OTHER FAST FACTS BOOKS

Fast Facts for the CATH LAB NURSE *(McCulloch)*

Fast Facts About NEUROCRITICAL CARE: A Quick Reference for the Advanced Practice Provider *(McLaughlin)*

Fast Facts for DNP ROLE DEVELOPMENT: A Career Navigation Guide *(Menonna-Quinn, Tortorella Genova)*

Fast Facts for DEMENTIA CARE: What Nurses Need to Know in a Nutshell *(Miller)*

Fast Facts for HEALTH PROMOTION IN NURSING: Promoting Wellness in a Nutshell *(Miller)*

Fast Facts for STROKE CARE NURSING: An Expert Care Guide, Second Edition *(Morrison)*

Fast Facts for MAKING THE MOST OF YOUR CAREER IN NURSING *(Redulla)*

Fast Facts for the MEDICAL OFFICE NURSE: What You Really Need to Know in a Nutshell *(Richmeier)*

Fast Facts for the PEDIATRIC NURSE: An Orientation Guide in a Nutshell *(Rupert, Young)*

Fast Facts About FORENSIC NURSING: What You Need to Know *(Scannell)*

Fast Facts About the GYNECOLOGICAL EXAM: A Professional Guide for NPs, PAs, and Midwives, Second Edition *(Secor, Fantasia)*

Fast Facts About MEDICAL CANNABIS AND OPIOIDS: Minimizing Opioid Use Through Cannabis *(Smith, Smith)*

Fast Facts for the STUDENT NURSE: Nursing Student Success in a Nutshell *(Stabler-Haas)*

Fast Facts About RELIGION FOR NURSES: Implications for Patient Care *(Taylor)*

Fast Facts for CAREER SUCCESS IN NURSING: Making the Most of Mentoring in a Nutshell *(Vance)*

Fast Facts for the TRIAGE NURSE: An Orientation and Care Guide, Second Edition *(Visser, Montejano)*

Fast Facts for the CLINICAL NURSE LEADER *(Wilcox, Deerhake)*

Fast Facts for DEVELOPING A NURSING ACADEMIC PORTFOLIO: What You Really Need to Know in a Nutshell *(Wittmann-Price)*

Fast Facts for the HOSPICE NURSE: A Concise Guide to End-of-Life Care *(Wright)*

Fast Facts for the CLASSROOM NURSING INSTRUCTOR: Classroom Teaching in a Nutshell *(Yoder-Wise, Kowalski)*

Forthcoming FAST FACTS Books

Fast Facts for NURSE PRACTITIONERS: Practice Essentials for Clinical Subspecialties *(Aktan)*

Fast Facts for the ER NURSE: Guide to a Successful Emergency Department Orientation, Fourth Edition *(Buettner)*

Fast Facts for the ADULT-GERONTOLOGY ACUTE CARE NURSE PRACTITIONER *(Carpenter)*

Fast Facts for WRITING THE DNP PROJECT: Eff ective Structure, Content, and Presentation *(Christenbery)*

Fast Facts for the NURSE PRECEPTOR: Keys to Providing a Successful Preceptorship, Second Edition *(Ciocco)*

Fast Facts for the NEONATAL NURSE: Care Essentials for Normal and High-Risk Neonates, Second Edition *(Davidson)*

Fast Facts about DIVERSITY, EQUITY, AND INCLUSION *(Davis)*

Fast Facts for the L&D NURSE: Labor & Delivery Orientation, Third Edition *(Groll)*

Fast Facts for the Radiology Nurse: An Orientation and Nursing Care Guide, Second Edition *(Grossman)*

Fast Facts for CREATING A SUCCESSFUL TELEHEALTH SERVICE: A How-to Guide for Nurse Practitioners *(Heidesch)*

Fast Facts for PATIENT SAFETY IN NURSING *(Hunt)*

Fast Facts for DEMENTIA CARE: What Nurses Need to Know, Second Edition *(Miller)*

Fast Facts for PEDIATRIC PRIMARY CARE: A Guide for Nurse Practitioners and Physician Assistants *(Ruggiero)*

Fast Facts About SEXUALLY TRANSMITTED INFECTIONS (STIs): A Nurse's Guide to Expert Patient Care *(Scannell)*

Fast Facts About LGBTQ CARE FOR NURSES *(Traister)*

Fast Facts About COMPETENCY-BASED EDUCATION IN NURSING: How to Teach Competency Mastery *(Wittmann-Price, Gittings)*

Fast Facts for the HOSPICE NURSE: A Concise Guide to End-of-Life Care, Second Edition *(Wright)*

Visit www.springerpub.com to order.

FAST FACTS for
MAKING THE MOST OF YOUR
CAREER IN NURSING

Rhoda R. Redulla, DNP, RN-BC, is the Magnet® Program Director at NewYork-Presbyterian/Weill Cornell Medical Center, a Magnet-designated, top five hospital in the United States. She previously served as the Director of Nursing Practice and Magnet Program Director at the Hospital of University of Pennsylvania. Dr. Redulla is an innovative nurse leader and is passionate about mentoring and inspiring nurses to achieve their full potential. Through various leadership roles, she has successfully spearheaded nursing fellowship programs, led the redesign of a nursing professional practice model, and championed the implementation of nursing peer review, competency assessment, and professional governance—key elements of the American Nurses Credentialing Center (ANCC) Magnet Recognition Program®.

Dr. Redulla has authored and coauthored books and book chapters in gastroenterology nursing, and she has also authored peer-reviewed articles. She is an evidence summary writer for Cochrane Nursing and a Certified Systematic Reviewer for the Joanna Briggs Institute, an international organization focused on evidence-based healthcare, based in Adelaide, Australia. Dr. Redulla has presented in national and international forums on Magnet, professional development, and management of hepatitis C. Most recently, she was an invited speaker at the Nursing Times Directors' Congress, Nursing Times Careers Live, and World Health Organization/Public Health England Conference. Dr. Redulla also chairs the Society of Gastroenterology Nurses and Associates (SGNA) Education Committee and is an expert reviewer for the *American Journal of Nursing and Gastroenterology Nursing.* She obtained her DNP degree from Johns Hopkins University and was named an outstanding alumna in 2019. She completed a post-master's certificate from the University of Pennsylvania and MA and BSN degrees from the University of Northern Philippines. She is nationally board certified in nursing professional development.

As an internationally educated nurse, Dr. Redulla is committed to promoting and supporting the professional development of nurse immigrants. She is an active member of the Philippine Nurses Association of America and Philippine Nurses Association of New Jersey and the founding president of its Gloucester County subchapter. In this book, she speaks about the value of being involved. Aside from her involvement in professional nursing organizations, Dr. Redulla is also a long-time volunteer of the Red Cross and her local church.

FAST FACTS for
MAKING THE MOST OF
YOUR CAREER IN NURSING

Rhoda R. Redulla, DNP, RN-BC

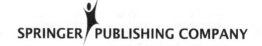

SPRINGER PUBLISHING COMPANY

Springer Publishing Company, LLC
11 West 42nd Street, New York, NY 10036
www.springerpub.com
connect.springerpub.com/

Acquisitions Editor: Joseph Morita
Compositor: Amnet Systems

ISBN: 978-0-8261-7314-0
ebook ISBN: 978-0-8261-7315-7
DOI: 10.1891/9780826173157

20 21 22 23 / 5 4 3 2 1

Library of Congress Cataloging-in-Publication Data

Names: Redulla, Rhoda, author, editor.
Title: Fast facts for making the most of your career in nursing / Rhoda
  Redulla.
Other titles: Fast facts (Springer Publishing Company)
Description: New York, NY : Springer Publishing Company, LLC, [2021] |
  Series: Fast facts | Includes bibliographical references and index.
Identifiers: LCCN 2020008183 (print) | LCCN 2020008184 (ebook) | ISBN
  9780826173140 (paperback) | ISBN 9780826173157 (ebook)
Subjects: MESH: Nursing | Staff Development
Classification: LCC RT82 (print) | LCC RT82 (ebook) | NLM WY 16.1 | DDC
  610.7306/9—dc23
LC record available at https://lccn.loc.gov/2020008183
LC ebook record available at https://lccn.loc.gov/2020008184

*To my wonderful husband, Tim, and my children, Tricia and Noah,
for inspiring me to be my best. Always.
To my parents and brother, Raymond, for being my first teachers.
To all nurses for whom this book is written: Thank you for making
the world a much better place.
In a special way, I dedicate this book to my amazing team at
NewYork-Presbyterian/Weill Cornell Medical Center.*

Contents

Contributors

Uvannie Enriquez, MPA, BSN, RN, NEA-BC
Patient Care Director
Weill Cornell Medical Center
NewYork-Presbyterian Hospital
New York, New York

Georgia Giannopoulos, MS, RD-AP, SHRM-CP, CDN, CNSC
Manager of Health and Wellbeing
NewYork-Presbyterian Hospital
New York, New York

Rhoda R. Redulla, DNP, RN-BC
Magnet® Program Director
Weill Cornell Medical Center
NewYork-Presbyterian Hospital
New York, New York

Lisa Roman-Fischetti, MSN, RN, NEA-BC
Magnet® Program Manager
Children's Hospital of Philadelphia
Philadelphia, Pennsylvania

Avis M. Russ, MBA, MS, BSN, RN, NE-BC
Magnet® Program Director
Westchester Division & NYP/Weill Cornell Psychiatry Program
NewYork-Presbyterian Hospital
New York, New York

Peter Stoffan, MPA, BSN, RN, CCRN, NEA-BC
Patient Care Director
NewYork Presbyterian Hospital
New York, New York

Carolyn Sun, PhD, RN, ANP-BC
Assistant Professor
Hunter College
Nurse Researcher/Nurse Scientist
NewYork-Presbyterian Hospital
New York, New York

Patricia Toth, DNP, RN, CHSE
Simulation Educator
Penn Medicine Clinical Simulation Center
Penn Medicine at Rittenhouse
Philadelphia, Pennsylvania

Success Story Contributors

Rita K. Adeniran, DrNP, RN, NEA-BC, FNAP, FAAN
Kathy A. Baker, PhD, APRN, ACNS-BC, FAAN
Joanne Bosanquet, MBE, RN
Ophelia M. Byers, DNP, RN, WHNP-BC, RNC-OB, NEA-BC
Cara Davis, MSN, RN, CCRN
Mary Ann Donohue-Ryan, PhD, RN, APN, PMH-CNS, NEA-BC, CPHQ
Elizabeth Froh, PhD, RN
Kelly Gallagher, MSN, RN-BC, NE-BC
Jason H. Gilbert, PhD, MBA, RN, NEA-BC
Kellyanne LaFrado, MSN, RN, CPN
Patrick Lallier, MPA, BSN, RN, CCRN
Janine Llamzon, MS, AGNPc, RN, CEN, NEA-BC
Maureen (Mickey) Mullin, MSN, RN, NEA-BC
Stephanie Nolan, DNP, MBA, RN, CPAN, NEA-BC
Stephanie O'Neill, BSN, RN
Suzanne Rubin, DNP, MPH, CRNP-P
Courtney Ruck, MSN, RN, SCRN
Daphne Stannard, PhD, RN-BC, CNS, FCCM
Carolyn Sun, PhD, RN, ANP-BC
Donna Zucker, PhD, RN, FAAN

Foreword

Nursing is a wonderful profession and a rewarding career, and never before have the possibilities for engagement been so diverse—from the bedside to the boardroom. Yet seizing the opportunities and optimizing your personal potential require thoughtful and intentional tactics and strategies. In many ways, the more opportunities presented to an individual, the more daunting career planning can be. *Fast Facts for Making the Most of Your Career in Nursing* provides a useful road map to optimize your career potential and provides tools to shape your career story. Your career story is in your hands, and your personal welfare and professional development should be strongly integrated. Engaging in and developing self-care plans and creating an identity beyond your role as a professional nurse are important. Good health, supportive relationships, and effective mentorship are integral to professional success and sustaining you through the good and bad times.

Developing goals and defining your legacy can be daunting. Your personal career journey will be one of ebbs and flows. Success, as you define it, doesn't happen passively or instantly—it happens when you show up, seize opportunities, make the connections, and truly own your story. Through proposing evocative questions, exemplars of success, and pragmatic tools to plan and strategize, *Fast Facts for Making the Most of Your Career in Nursing* is a useful tool for career planning and professional development.

Effective nurse leaders need to undertake a critical self-reflective appraisal of their strengths and weaknesses as part of a lifelong learning process, and this practice is integral to career development. Developing networks, competencies, and interpersonal skills is just as important for effectiveness as clinical competency. *Fast Facts for Making the Most of Your Career in Nursing* is a pragmatic text, drawing on pivotal leadership perspectives and embedded examples from successful nurses to provide to novice and experienced nurses both, a road map for professional growth. Redulla draws on her own rich professional journey to provide candid and moving examples from her career.

Fast Facts for Making the Most of Your Career in Nursing is being released at a critical time in the history of professional nursing. The year 2020 was named the Year of the Nurse and Midwife by the World Health Organization; we need to reflect on our successes as well as the challenges we have faced and continue to face on our professional journey. The year 2020 also marked the 200th anniversary of the birth of Florence Nightingale, who set the course of modern professional nursing. Nurses need to not only be caring and compassionate but also be abreast of scientific knowledge and be technically competent. We have come a long way and celebrate with pride being the most trusted professional group. But we still face many challenges, particularly in being allowed to practice to the top of our license and demonstrating our value proposition to funders and policy makers. In many regions of the country, the nursing workforce still does not reflect the diversity and heterogeneity of contemporary society. We also struggle to address social determinants of health and promote an agenda of social justice, diversity, equity, and inclusion.

To seize the opportunities presented to us and address the challenges ahead, we need to be prepared. *Fast Facts for Making the Most of Your Career in Nursing* will be a handbook for your entire career. Remember, the opportunities are endless, and you will need to seek supportive and enabling environments that will sustain your personal and professional career. I have been a nurse for over 40 years and have never for a moment regretted this career choice and have seized opportunities to work across a number of institutions. All the best for your future. Never before has our world needed competent, confident, and credentialed nurses to address the challenges we face. Never give up on nursing but work to find your niche and the motivation and support to drive you to do great work.

> *"Success is not final, failure is not fatal: It is the courage to continue that counts."*
>
> —Winston Churchill

Patricia M. Davidson, PhD, MED, RN, FAAN
Dean and Professor
Johns Hopkins School of Nursing
Baltimore, Maryland

Preface

One of the most profound lessons I have learned is "Never stagnate." This was the key message of our commencement speaker during my high school graduation. That was a long time ago, but it stuck with me through the years. This is the same advice I would have for every nurse. Never stagnate, regardless of the stage you are in, in your professional career.

Have you encountered a nursing living legend? How about an American Nurses Association (ANA) Hall of Famer? Have you ever wondered, "How did they do it?" Is there a magic bullet to achieving this professional success? Probably not. A huge dose of preparation and grit, that's for sure. For now, you may not be aspiring to be the next living legend of your generation. Most likely though, you are aiming to take that next step in your career. This book presents practical strategies on how you (nurses) can advance in your professional nursing journey. What are the options open to you as you pursue professional development opportunities? Where should you be looking for support? What could be holding you back from moving forward in your career? This book will serve as a how-to resource in making the most of your nursing career. Each chapter includes examples from nurses who experienced these roles firsthand, with specific advice on how to reach your full potential and even how to aim for things that are out of reach.

This book will be helpful to healthcare organizations in pursuing the American Nurses Credentialing Center (ANCC) Magnet® Recognition Program and Pathway to Excellence. Aligned with transformational leadership and structural empowerment, the book provides insight on how healthcare organizations can best support nurses in developing professionally.

MAIN THEMES AND OBJECTIVES

- To present the professional opportunities available to nurses at all levels
- To provide practical advice on how to navigate various professional development pathways and advance in the nursing journey
- To spark inspiration among nurses to be the best version of themselves and grow in their professional nursing careers

PEDAGOGICAL FEATURES

Success stories

- Feature successful nurses
- Highlight lessons from successful nurses

KEY POINTS

- Summary at the end of each chapter presented in bullet point format

KEY FEATURES OF THIS BOOK

- Provides nurses "a starting point" when they find themselves stuck in their professional nursing journey
- Both frontline nurses and nurse leaders will benefit from the resources and tools included in the book
- Creates a useful connection with the ANCC Magnet Recognition® and Pathway to Excellence® programs
- Provides advice to specific groups such as nurse immigrants and second-degree nurses, who go through unique pathways in professional development
- Uplifting success stories from nurses of diverse experience and expertise
- Each chapter opens with an inspiring quote from contributors

DESCRIPTION OF EACH CHAPTER

Chapter 1. Finding Your Why

Do you find yourself reflecting on what brings you fulfillment and helps you discover your purpose? Are you thinking of the changes you can make that can lead you to reach your full potential? Then this chapter is for you! It includes strategies and approaches to help you pursue that next step that will allow you to be your best self.

Chapter 2. Aspire and Achieve: Creating Your Professional Road Map

When was the last time you updated your curriculum vitae (CV) or résumé? What do you plan to do in the next 5 years? 10 years? The highlight of this chapter is conducting a professional gap analysis. A professional gap analysis encompasses asking the questions: Where am I now? Where do I wish I should be? and How do I close that gap? In this chapter, you will also learn to develop your CV and create your professional development plan.

Chapter 3. Embracing Opportunity

Remember the old adage "Opportunity knocks when you least expect it"? As Kathleen Ann Thompson, a renowned life coach and blogger, wrote, "Opportunity has already come knocking. And I didn't do much of anything." Well, this chapter will prepare you for that opportunity—to advance from a frontline clinical role to a nurse leader or to shift from the practice setting to academia, or even taking a huge leap to accept a promotion that involves a major relocation.

Chapter 4. Being Involved: What's in It for Me?

This chapter shows you the endless possibilities to be involved: within the organization, in a professional nursing organization, and in the community. If you ask me, I am who I am now professionally largely because I have been involved in projects and organizations beyond my regular scope of work.

Chapter 5. Making a Difference in Research, Evidence-Based Practice, and Quality Improvement

This chapter continues the theme of how you can be involved, with concentration on quality improvement, evidence-based practice, and research. It also shows you an important step in any improvement work: dissemination. You will get practical advice on how you can disseminate your work effectively through scholarly presentations, publications, podcasts, and social media.

Chapter 6. Seeking Your Mentor

Do you have a favorite mentor? Or have you been a mentor to another colleague? This chapter includes strategies on how to initiate and develop a relationship with a mentor. It also includes the benefits of successful mentorship.

Chapter 7. Becoming an Expert

Patricia Benner clearly demonstrated the five stages of proficiency, more widely known as "from novice to expert." This chapter presents how nurses become experts through academic progression and by pursuing professional nursing certification. It provides specific advice on selecting an academic program, how to apply, eligibility for national nursing specialty certification, and how to prepare for the examination.

Chapter 8. Embracing a New Culture

This chapter provides a special focus on the transition of internationally educated nurses and nurse immigrants as new professionals in a new country, and includes helpful advice in nurturing their professional growth. It touches on the struggles of nurse immigrants as they assimilate into a new culture while developing as a professional. The chapter highlights strategies on how to conquer these challenges and features the lived experience of three successful nurse immigrants.

Chapter 9. Nursing as a Second Career

Second-career nurse or not, you will love and learn a ton from this chapter. The author, Peter Stoffan, completed a musical theater degree prior to being a nurse. He outlines his advice to nurses in an engaging letter format. This chapter takes you to a deeper level of understanding and appreciation for those pursuing nursing as a second career. The incredible success stories in this chapter feature how nurses discovered fulfillment in their new professional path.

Chapter 10. Effective Networking

This chapter presents strategies on effective networking and showcases successful nurses who made the most of this professional development strategy. When you think networking is just about meeting people, you could be wrong. It involves creating a meaningful connection with colleagues, establishing a relationship, and nurturing it.

Chapter 11. Self-Care for Nurses

This chapter is about you and what you can do to nurture your mind, body, and spirit. I am uniquely excited about this chapter. I partnered with Georgia Giannopoulos, an advanced practice registered dietitian, to complete this chapter. This includes self-care ideas and how nurses can make this happen. It also includes helpful resources tailored for nurses and how can organizations support self-care for their teams.

Chapter 12. Career Opportunities for Nurses

Have you read the book *301 Careers in Nursing?* You will be amazed about the almost endless role possibilities and opportunities for nurses. This chapter presents these career opportunities and helpful advice on how to get there.

Rhoda R. Redulla

Acknowledgments

I grew up and started my nursing career in the Philippines. I would have never imagined that someday, I would be writing my own book about making the most of your nursing career. This work is an absolute dream come true and has been one of the most rewarding experiences in my career. I am especially thrilled that this book will be launched in the International Year of the Nurse. None of these would have been possible without the support and love of my family. To my husband, Tim, my pillar and best friend. You were the first person who encouraged me to submit my first conference abstract many moons ago. To my children, Tricia and Noah, you are a bundle of love, and you are a gift in every way. You constantly remind me that there is always something to be grateful for—and to laugh about. Thank you for being patient and quiet during long car rides, just so I could wrap up another section of the book. To my parents, Lito and Francisca, my brother, Raymond, and his family, and the rest of my family in the Philippines—your unconditional love keeps me going through good days and hard ones.

A special thank you to all the amazing chapter authors. You embraced this opportunity to be part of the book with unbelievable enthusiasm and delivered excellence in every page you wrote. You gave 101%—from coming up with practical advice to pursuing the best evidence to conducting interviews.

To the success story contributors, I can't wait to see the many nurses who will be inspired by your incredible commitment to nursing and drive to elevate the status of nurses.

A heartfelt thank you to Dr. Patricia Davidson, dean, Johns Hopkins University School of Nursing. What an incredible honor to have you write the foreword.

To my New York-Presbyterian family, most especially to my nursing team. You are the inspiration behind this book! Special thanks to VP and Chief Nursing Officer Rosanne Raso and Dr. Beverly Karas-Irwin, my two bosses, whose guidance and mentorship are second to none. To Chief Nurse Executive and Chief Quality Officer Wilhelmina Manzano and Vice President for Nursing Operations MariLou Prado-Inzerillo, thank you for your inspiring leadership.

To my mentors when I was a young professional back home in the Philippines (Drs. Ferdinand Lamarca, Ocarna Figuerres, Lauro Tacbas, Salvador Eder, and Julia Amigable), UNP College of Nursing family, my mentors at Penn Medicine (Drs. Gregory Ginsberg, Thomas Faust, Nuzhat Ahmad, Michael Kochman, and Victoria Rich), and the Society of Gastroenterology Nurses and Associates (Drs. Kathy Baker, Donna Zucker, Sharon Dudley-Brown, and Cindy Friis). To Dr. Mary Terhaar and my DNP faculty mentors, I will always cherish my Hopkins education as a remarkable gift and privilege.

To my former team at Penn Medicine, most especially in nursing professional development and the GI/Hepatology Division, I have spent the best years growing as a nursing professional with you.

To nursing colleagues Pam Mack-Brooks, Rita Adeniran, Pat Smith, Cynthia Richardson, Hazel Bambalan, Madelyn Yu, Suzanne Rubin, Amanda Mastrangelo, Janet Zimmerman, Kathleen O'Shea, Rose McGonigle, and Carol Endozo. You have touched my life as a nurse in the most profound way.

To family and friends who help me and my family in our life's journey: Faith Duran, Rizalio and Joy Manigsaca, Bayawa, Sayson, Vargas, Montero, Bautista, Perales, and Couples for Christ families.

To the Springer Publishing Company editors Joe Morita and Hannah Hicks and the entire Springer nursing team. I love working with you! Thank you for your exceptional guidance and keen insight from conception to completion of the book.

Lastly, to God, from whom all goodness flows.

1

Finding Your Why

Carolyn Sun and Rhoda R. Redulla

"If you don't know where you're going, any road will take you there."
—Bill George

You just got to work: Do you know your goal for today? Will today be a repeat of yesterday? Without a clear vision of what you aim to accomplish in the short term and long term, today will seem like yesterday. And the next day, and the next day. This is a book about how to advance your professional nursing career, but before you can begin to do that, it is important to reflect on what it is that is driving you to advance your career. Is it to make more money? To have a more flexible schedule so you can spend time with your family? What is it that drives you? In this chapter, we set the stage by helping you to think about what it is that drives you—your "why."

WHY IS IT IMPORTANT TO KNOW YOUR WHY?

By knowing your why, you become more deliberate in your choices and actions from day to day. If you have a clear vision of your future and purpose, both personally and professionally, chances are you will be more successful. Just like you wouldn't try to go somewhere you had never been without directions to get there, it's difficult to plan to advance your career without an end goal in mind and a plan about how you might get there. You might be lucky and get there by accident, but more often than not, having a game plan will ensure that you arrive at your destination more quickly. In his famous book, *The Seven Habits of Highly Effective People*, Steven Covey sets forth the tenet "Begin with the End in Mind" (Covey, 1989). He states,

> *"People are working harder than ever, but because they lack clarity and vision, they aren't getting very far. They, in essence, are pushing a rope with all of their might."*
>
> —Dr. Stephen Covey

Where is it you would like to go? Many of us do not have a clear idea about this; that is to say, we know that we'd like to be able to retire at some point, to be happy, to be healthy, to not have to worry about money, to have a schedule that suits our lifestyle, and so forth, but we are unclear about what it takes to achieve those things. By outlining what matters to you, you can begin to see what kinds of jobs you would be happiest doing because you can also think about what it would take to have that job.

For example, if I want to be the chief nursing officer of my organization, I know that I will be able to have financial security and early retirement. But I will also have to put in tons of long, hard hours and be willing to work nights and weekends. You may have heard the saying "Work smarter not harder." That is what we will do here; instead of diving headfirst into "being successful," we will think through where it is we want to go so that the steps we take will lead us there. This chapter will take some time and effort on your part, but it is a very important first step in the process of achieving success.

> *"Know thyself; γνῶθι σεαυτόν; gnōthi seauton."*
>
> —Ancient Greek Maxim

It is worth considering carefully what it is you *really* want. Sometimes we think we know, but oftentimes we can be good at lying to ourselves or really not knowing until we experience it. Growing up, I (CS) thought that once I had kids, I would like to stop working. When I met my husband, this was a source of conflict for us. He was sure that I was succumbing to cultural expectations rather than what would truly make me happy. When I had my first baby, I tried to stay home from work. It turned out he was absolutely right. I enjoyed my work immensely, and even though I loved being with my daughter, I missed my job. I had to reexamine myself and learn that what I thought about myself didn't match with who I was in reality.

Similarly, before I became a nurse, I was a graphic designer. It was my dream job as a kid and the one that I thought I would love, but I quickly found out that there were many aspects I didn't like. I felt my art came from my soul, and having people critique and change it really bothered me. I also didn't like having to be in an office just so that people could see my face; I wanted autonomy. I wanted the flexibility of being able to work from home, I wanted to travel, I wanted to do something creative but not have it be something that would break my heart if people didn't love it. In the end, I realized I wanted to be a scientist. I could design my own studies (tapping into the creative part of my brain) but not feel bad if people critiqued them. I could travel to present my work, and I could often work from home. The hours are long, but I love what I do, so it doesn't feel like work, and often I can do the work whenever and wherever I want. It took me a long time to figure out what I wanted to do, and it may take you a long time too, but I think if I had been more honest with myself up front, the road getting here might have been much shorter.

Make a list. What are the things driving you: Success? Autonomy? Power? Money? Having more time? Freedom? Recognition? What are absolute deal breakers: Being away from family? Working weekends? Ethical dilemmas? This last one may sound out of place—after all, you're already a nurse and maybe even chose nursing because of its noble reputation—but let's take some time to think this through.

COGNITIVE DISSONANCE?

Peter Drucker, father of modern American management, advised leaders to develop a deep understanding of their values and avoid or leave work situations that create cognitive dissonance (Sherman, 2017).

A friend of mine (CS) took an executive nursing job in the United Arab Emirates that paid an incredible amount of money—the salary was almost an unimaginable sum. The description seemed perfectly aligned with what she wanted to do, and all she had to do was move to Dubai. But once she was there, she had to work night and day—she had no personal freedom and was expected to be available all hours of the day and night. The cultural differences were more than she expected, and throughout the term of her contract, she felt trapped, but she could not break the terms of her contract and had to see it through.

Another friend of mine wanted to take a part-time job so she could spend more time with her family after giving birth. She was hired at a women's health clinic, where, among other things, she was expected to assist with abortions. At that time in her life, it was just unthinkable to her, and even though she loved most aspects of the job, she had to quit.

Both of these are extreme examples, but they help us to think about what kinds of situations we are willing to put ourselves in for things like money, freedom, or more time. Continue your list and reflect on what you *need* from a job, what you *hope* for in your career.

To help yourself identify what those values that drive you might be, think of a time when you've come across a dilemma in your professional nursing journey. Ask yourself these three questions:

- Was my decision congruent with my values?
- Was my action aligned with my beliefs?
- Was my decision consistent with my principles?

For each of these, reflect on why or why not. What was the decision or action you chose? What was the value, belief, or principle that made you respond in that way?

HOW TO FIND YOUR WHY: IS THERE AN APP FOR THAT?

In the digital world we are in now, perhaps sometimes you might be wondering is there a way, similar to a Google map, that helps you determine your professional road map? Let's say you are thinking of becoming a nurse educator, or a director of nursing research, or a wound and ostomy care nurse. Can you input your "desired destination," and the "app" suggests several possible routes to get there? That sounds amazing, doesn't it? In reality, you and I know very well that such an app does not exist. Every nurse or professional has unique circumstances that define their professional track. While there may not be an app to tell us what our personal journey should be, there may be some concrete steps we can take to help us begin to develop our own road map.

In 2007 Bill George published a highly successful book on authentic leadership called *Discover Your True North*. In his book, Mr. George suggests that in order to be a good leader, one must know themselves. What struck me (RR) was learning that true north is derived from most deeply held values, beliefs, and principles, and it can serve as an internal compass that helps guide you when your values are tested. Mr. George has graciously allowed us to reprint here a guide that he developed to help you discover your true north.

DISCOVERING YOUR TRUE NORTH (BILL GEORGE, 30 QUESTIONS)

30 questions to help you find your True North. Don't answer them all at once. Take a day to carefully think each one through. Remember, if you don't know where you're going, any road will take you there.

1. What you want your legacy to be? 10, 20, 50 years from now, what will your name mean? [What do you like about this question? What is tough about this question?]

2. What one word do you want people to use to describe you? What do you think they'd currently use?

3. If money was no object, how would you spend your time? What would your day look like?

4. Fill in the blank: My life is a quest for _____. What motivates you? Money? Love? Acceptance?

5. If you were to donate everything you have to a cause or charity, which would it be?

6. What is your biggest regret? If you could go back and have a "redo," what would you change?

7. When was the last time you told a lie? Why? What would have happened if you had told the truth?

8. If you accomplish one thing by the end of the year, what would make the biggest impact on your happiness?

9. What do you think is the meaning of life? Do you live your life accordingly?

10. What would others say is your biggest asset? What would they say is your biggest flaw? Be honest.

11. What did you like to do when you were 10 years old? When was the last time you did that activity?

12. What do you love most about your current job? What do you wish you could do more of?

13. What do you think you were put on this earth to learn? What were you put here to teach?

14. What keeps you awake at night when you should be sleeping? What gets you out of bed in the mornings?

15. List your core values. Use your company's mission statement to list its core values. Do they match up?

16. What skills do people frequently compliment you on? These may not be what you think you're best at.

17. If you had the opportunity to get a message across to a large group of people, what would you say?

18. What do you not want others to know about you? Use your answer to find and conquer insecurities.

19. List the five people you interact with most frequently (not necessarily friends). How is each helping you to reach your goals (or not)?

20. If yourself from 10 years ago met you today, would he/she be impressed with where you've gotten? Why or why not?

21. What bugs you? If it makes you mad, you're passionate about it! Can you make your anger productive?

22. Fast-forward 10 or 20 years. What is the one thing that, if you never pursued it, you'd always regret?

23. When was the last time you embarrassed yourself? You have to be vulnerable to find your purpose.

24. Who or what energizes you? What makes you feel depleted? Do you thrive on chaos or prefer order?

25. Who do you look up to? Who are your mentors, both those you know personally and those who inspire you from afar?
26. Think about your talents, passions, and values. How can you use them to serve and contribute to society?
27. Why do you want to find your purpose? Write the answer down and put it somewhere you can see it. The journey isn't always easy.
28. What in your life is "on hold"? Until you lose weight, until you retire, etc. What are you waiting for?
29. What price would you take to give up on your dreams? What price would you be willing to pay to achieve them?
30. Now that you've answered these questions, what is your action plan? What steps will you take today? Let's look at a real-life success story. (George, 2015)

SUCCESS STORY

Mary Ann Donohue-Ryan, PhD, RN, APN, PMH-CNS, NEA-BC, CPHQ

Executive Consultant, Chilton Medical Center, Atlantic Health System, Pompton Lakes, NJ

Describe your professional nursing journey, including your current role.

As a newly minted registered nurse, I believed in three things: the value of education; being blessed with the gifts of stamina, drive, and determination; and, most importantly, my family and their unwavering support and belief in my success even when I did not always see my future path ahead of me.

I began as a staff nurse at the same hospital that was attached to my diploma school of nursing. I was very emotionally attached to this hospital, having also volunteered there all throughout high school and worked in the Admissions Office every weekend in nursing school. After I graduated, the biggest challenge at the time was adjusting to the rigors of simultaneous university study, working in the ED, and acclimating to the psychosocial climate of the hospital environment. There was a distinct anti-education bias among my fellow nurses, and it was very unusual at the time for someone to attend BSN classes by day/evening and working the night shift as a newly graduated nurse. My strong beliefs in education as a vehicle to personal and professional improvement, however, was unshakable. Once in the classroom, I soaked up every lecture and applied the content to my overall level of knowledge about patient care, and thought about how my own contributions at the unit level as well as how my future career would be professionally impacted. I was addicted to books; to journal articles; to my professional organization, New Jersey State Nurses Association (NJSNA), and the American Nurses Association (ANA), which I joined as soon as I learned about it; to local and national nursing leaders; and to the idea that I was going to graduate school for my master's degree and my doctoral degree as soon as possible. In that RN-to-baccalaureate program, I developed relationships with other like-minded nurses who were advancing educationally. It was still difficult to come to the hospital workplace where I had attended diploma school and had so much history, yet I soaked up valuable lessons from the more seasoned nurses and attribute so many life lessons to my first years as a nurse there.

What are one or two pieces of advice that you can share for new nurses as they embark on "finding their why"? How can nurses reach their full potential?

Three things:

1. Ambition, stamina, and an insatiable sense of curiosity beat out natural intelligence every time and every day. I was not the smartest person in my class in nursing school; any professional achievements in my life were hard won.
2. Always remember why you became a nurse in the first place and reconcile the "bad" days with what characteristics were clearly and not-so-clearly missing from that particular day, experience, or interaction.
3. Don't put your professional eggs in one basket. By that I mean, do not expect that one nursing unit, one supervisor, one coworker, or even one hospital organization will meet your broad professional needs for your whole life, nor will that define you, unless you let it. You must get involved in your professional organization and move beyond simple dues-paying. Leadership behaviors are developed and nurtured in professional organizations, and this is crucial if every nurse is to be a leader to advocate for their patients at the frontline level of care. From my early days as a district/region #2 volunteer to president of the New Jersey State Nurses Association, I am proud to work alongside staff nurses.

What are you most proud of, professionally?

As a leader, I'm most proud that all my efforts are always directed at the frontline level of care delivery. For example, I know that when I've made weekend/holiday rounds, and the staff have been at first, surprised and pleased to see me and to engage with me about their interactions that particular shift or they have called or texted me about a challenge or a success, then I know I have been a truthful, accessible, and genuine leader to them.

As a Magnet® leader, I am very proud that I contributed to two of the first nine standards in the early 1990s that resulted in the inaugural American Nurses Credentialing Center (ANCC) Magnet standards. It was a sincere thrill that I will never forget, that I created the first Magnet gap analysis template, and, along with other nurse leaders at the first Magnet hospital, submitted the first Magnet application after the pilot organization. Becoming the second Magnet hospital in the country and the accompanying media coverage were moments in my shared history that will never be forgotten.

Our chief nursing officer at the time supported me to be named to the ANCC Governing Body at the Institute for Credentialing International, where I had the honor of serving under Dr. Margretta Madden Styles, Dr. Patricia Yoder-Wise, and so many others. As a member of that group, my contributions have been acknowledged in research journals (Cheung & Aiken, 2006; Kramer et al., 2007) and in quality journals (Lundmark & Hickey, 2007) and in a textbook (Barker, Sullivan, & Emery, 2006).

My interest and passion has always been to educate others about the Magnet journey to excellence since the early days, when an organization's Magnet designation was thought to be proprietary, and, thus, not to be shared. I suppose I broke the rules, because I shared and educated on my own time as necessary. I have traveled locally, nationally, and internationally (United Kingdom and Singapore), leading to numerous organizations' first Magnet designations. As a nursing director, I've led my first organization to its first four Magnet designations; as a chief nursing officer, I've led three Magnet designations in two separate organizations. I am certified in the Fundamentals of Magnet by the American Nurses Credentialing Center (ANCC), as an adult psychiatric-mental health clinical nurse specialist, and a nurse executive, advanced, through the ANCC. I am also certified as a certified professional in healthcare quality (CPHQ) by the National Association of Healthcare Quality.

Since the journey to excellence is just that, a journey and not a destination in and of itself, the Magnet model and standards are the worthiest guidance one can utilize as a professional leader.

LEARNING BY EXAMPLE

We have spent a lot of time up front thinking about what it is that drives us and figuring out something about who we are as a person. Now, let's use this success story as a case study for what can make us successful. From this example, we see that Dr. Donohue-Ryan had a deep belief that education was important. She knew herself—her stamina, drive, and determination—and her resources—her family's support. We also read that even as a diploma nurse, she used the experiences and relationships she had professionally to develop her career. Her love for learning drove her to read everything she could get her hands on.

We can see that some of these are internal resources—things that come from within Dr. Donohue-Ryan that help to ensure her success—her determination, her hardworking nature, and her drive. I (CS) have to take a moment to say how deeply I agree with Dr. Donohue-Ryan about the importance of stamina. Most of the smartest and most successful people I know will say they are not that smart; they just are determined. A really successful friend and colleague told me that growing up, her dad always told her, "We aren't the smartest people, so we have to put in twice as many hours." I disagree, she is definitely one of the smartest people I know, but she also puts in the hours like no one else I know. I have watched her success grow over the years—everyone sees that she will put in any amount of time to get the job done well. Think about what internal resources you have: Is it your drive? Your faith? Your patience? Or maybe you really are the smartest person. Whatever it is, make a little table like Table 1.1, and write it down. Hang it up and look at it every day. Remind yourself of all the things you have going for you—your friends, your intelligence, your drive. I can tell already that you are brilliant and determined. Who else would take the time to read this book? Write those down in the "internal resources" column.

Table 1.1

Sorting Out My Resources Using the Success Story Example

What Drives Me (My Why)?	What Are My *Internal* Resources to Achieve My Goals?	What Are My *External* Resources to Achieve My Goals?
Example:		
■ Importance of education for myself and for my vocational success	■ Stamina ■ Drive ■ Determination ■ Insatiable sense of curiosity	■ Family support ■ Professional experiences ■ Professional relationships
Write in your own answers here:		
■	■	■
■	■	■
■	■	■

Others are resources that are external—her family support, the relationship with her colleagues, and her professional experiences. You may not have money, but you might have access to scholarships, a great support network, contacts in high places, and so on. Even if you think you don't have any of those things, let me tell you that you do. If you put in a little bit of elbow grease, you can accomplish almost anything. Let me give you an example.

Once, when I was living in Seattle, I went to see a movie with a few of my nurse friends from work, and during the credits, we saw a name credited and the position they were listed as having was "set nurse." From that moment on, I made it my personal life goal to work on a film set. Later, I moved to New York City to get my master's degree. While I was in school, I found out that my clinical instructor worked at National Broadcasting Company (NBC) Universal, so I asked if she would precept me for some of my clinical hours. She said she couldn't because she was new to the position and scared about having too many things going on because it was a really busy clinic. I promised her that if she took me, I would only help relieve her workload and wouldn't be a nuisance. She continued to politely decline, and I continued to pester her until she finally relented. Once I got there, I pretended as if I were running for president. I would say hello and smile to every single person I met and tried hard to remember their names (sometimes I would bump into celebrities in the hallway and say hello as if we were old friends, before I realized who they were). I would do any job that no one wanted to do, and lots of jobs people hadn't even thought of (cleaning the exam rooms, the equipment, restocking before things were empty, etc.). When I finished my clinical rotation, I asked if they'd be willing to hire me as a per diem nurse. And they did! Once they hired me as a nurse, I asked if they would hire me as a nurse practitioner when I graduated from school—they did. I continued to work hard and do any and every job they had for me even as I went on to pursue my doctorate degree, and even when it was inconvenient for me. I had a newborn and toddler at home, and I think I made less from the job than it cost me to hire a babysitter. One day when I was walking back from lunch at school, I got a call asking if I would be willing to be a set nurse for *Saturday Night Live*. For me, it was a dream come true! This is kind of a silly example (obviously there are much more highly regarded jobs and much more important kinds of work than working on a TV set), but I think it demonstrates how things can happen if you (a) have a clear goal of what you want to do, (b) don't give up on that goal, and (c) work hard to get there. When I share this story with my most successful friends, each of them has a similar story of doggedly pursuing their dreams until they came true.

It's also good to remember that sometimes things are not as far out of reach as they seem. For instance, when we were writing this chapter, RR wanted to include the questionnaire from Bill George, so she reached out to him via email, and he gave permission immediately. Wow! A famous author gives permission in just one afternoon. Pretty amazing. Perhaps people are nicer than we think.

Going back to our exemplar, although she didn't state what her goals were early on (other than getting an education), we see from what makes her most proud that her goal probably included being a truthful, accessible, and genuine leader—which she achieved. Maybe you can reverse engineer your goals the same way (Table 1.2). Look at the lists and checklist that you completed in the previous sections. By looking at what you would do, if you could, and by thinking about what makes you most proud, or what makes you most uncomfortable, you may be able to shake out what are your true goals in life and in your professional career. In other chapters of this book, we talk about the specific professional mechanisms by which those goals might be accomplished, but figuring out the deeper values and meaning behind them is much more difficult and much more important.

Table 1.2

Reverse Engineering My Goals: Example From the Success Story	
What Makes Me the Proudest?	**Goals**
Examples from the story: Becoming the second Magnet* hospital in the country	Recognition of hard work
My efforts are always directed at the frontline level of care delivery	Improving patient care
When the staff have been, at first, surprised and pleased to see me and to engage with me about their interactions that particular shift or they have called or texted me about a challenge or a success	To be a truthful, accessible, and genuine leader
Write in your own answers here:	

PUTTING IT ALL TOGETHER

Throughout this chapter, we've been writing down answers to questions and spending time delving into things. At this point, we have thought through:

1. What drives you (values)
2. Cognitive dissonance (what you are unwilling to do)
3. Your internal resources
4. Your external resources
5. Goals

When you put all of these things together, you will have a much clearer idea of what you want, how you can achieve it, and what will bring you a good work–life balance. It might be helpful to visualize what this balance means (Figure 1.1). Your career is supported by

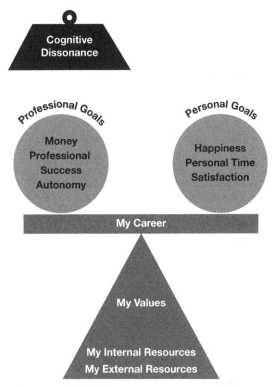

Figure 1.1 Creating work–life balance.
Source: Courtesy of Carolyn Sun.

your resources, and your career should help you reach these goals. Some may be professional goals, such as earning a good salary, being successful, and having autonomy. Others may be personal goals, such as having time for family or hobbies and achieving personal happiness. This balance is threatened by cognitive dissonance. Your personal values should support, guide, and balance your career and your professional and personal goals.

CHOOSE EXCELLENCE

> "There are many reasons to try and do great work rather than just 'good enough' work: It sets you apart from the rest of the pack. It makes people around you happier. It makes you happier. It's incredibly fun and satisfying.
>
> "But most of all, what else are you going to do with your life? What better thing to do with your time on earth than trying your hardest to make the world around you better? Imagine the world we'd live in if everyone did this. It starts with you."
>
> —Jamal Nichols (www.truthaboutdesign.com)

You could have decided to just pursue whatever you wanted to do without reading this book. Instead, you decided to read it. You decided to spend some time thinking about things, examining yourself, and coming up with a plan for how you will get there. You could have decided to do it all halfway—to skim the pages, to just go with the flow, and do whatever comes your way. But you didn't—you decided to choose greatness, as the saying goes. But let's change that; let's take it a step further. Choose excellence. My (CS) favorite proverb is:

> "Whatever your hand finds to do, do it with all your might."
>
> —Ecclesiastes 9:10

As I have moved into more of a leadership role over the years, what I have noticed time and again is that those who just put in that little bit of extra—those are the true standouts. Go beyond average; be excellent. As you continue to read this book and discover new paths to a successful professional nursing career, keep this in mind: Choose excellence.

Key Points

- Invest in carefully thinking about what you really want to do, what inspires you, and what gives you happiness.
- Knowing your true north and purpose propels you to achieve your fullest potential.
- Whatever you choose to do, do your best; choose excellence.

References

Barker, A. M., Sullivan, D. T., & Emery, M. J. (2006). *Leadership competencies for clinical managers: The renaissance of transformational leadership.* Sudbury, MA: Jones and Bartlett Publishers.

Cheung, R., & Aiken, L. H. (2006). Hospital initiatives to support a better-educated workforce. *Journal of Nursing Administration, 36*(7), 357–362. doi:10.1097/00005110-200607000-00007

Covey, S. R. (1989). *The 7 habits of highly effective people: Powerful lessons in personal change.* Lucerne, Switzerland: GetAbstract.

George, B. (2015, April 3). *30 Questions to help you discover your true north* [blog]. Retrieved from https://www.billgeorge.org/articles/30-questions-to-help-you-discover-your-true-north/

Kramer, M., Maguire, P., Schmalenberg, C. E., Andrews, B., Burke, R., Chmielewski, L. M., . . . Tachibana, C. (2007). Excellence through evidence: Structures enabling clinical autonomy. *Journal of Nursing Administration, 37*(1), 41–52. doi:10.1097/00005110-200701000-00007

Lundmark, V. A., & Hickey, J. V. (2007). The Magnet Recognition Program®: Developing a National Magnet Research Agenda. *Journal of Nursing Care Quality, 22*(3), 195–198. doi:10.1097/01.NCQ.0000277773.04901.53

Sherman, R. O. (2017). Finding your true north. *Nurse Leader, 15*(6), 370–371. doi:10.1016/j.mnl.2017.08.003

2

Aspire and Achieve: Creating Your Professional Road Map

Rhoda R. Redulla

"Every job I pursued in nursing always seemed to build upon previous experiences, making my practice (and my life) much fuller because of the diversity in roles and settings I experienced."
—Kathy Baker, PhD, ACNS, FAAN

One critical element to a successful career in nursing is an early, integrated exposure to research, education, and clinical practice (Hickey, 2018). Nurses use as many resources as possible to ensure they achieve this goal. Doing so involves taking advantage of diverse training opportunities, being exposed to research and evidence-based practice, and receiving expert mentorship in different areas (Hickey, 2018). I saw a nursing career billboard that showed: "Nursing, how you want to do it, when you want to do it, where you want to do it." The line is very empowering and encouraging. It conveys a strong message that you have the absolute power to create your own professional road map. First, how do you do it? The first step is a self-assessment to reflect on where you are on your career trajectory, your skill set, strengths, opportunities for growth, priorities, and your vision.

SELF-ASSESSMENT

A SWOT (strengths, weaknesses, opportunities, threats) analysis is a strategy commonly used in strategic planning for organizations. SWOT is also applicable for self-assessment and personal and professional goal setting (Tables 2.1 and 2.2). An important aspect of doing a SWOT analysis is purpose. Why are you doing it? Are you looking for a new job, new accomplishment, or just looking for change (Martin, 2015)? As you respond to these questions, think of your career goals.

Strengths

First, think of your strengths, not only in your current role or organization, but overall. Include accomplishments that you have not even thought about recently. Martin (2015) recommends asking yourself these questions:

- What are you good at naturally?

I have a colleague who is naturally inclined to enjoy process maps, fish bone diagrams, and root cause analysis. You can make a good guess on her professional role. She works as a nurse coordinator in quality and patient safety. Another former coworker is passionate about sharing her skills with others and always volunteers to orient new members of the team. She now works as a clinical instructor in a local community college. How about you? What do you love doing? Include these on your "strengths" list.

- What skills have you worked to develop?

Whether it is psychomotor, communication, or leadership skills, a few things will stand out as you reflect on your strengths. In clinical care, an example that easily comes to mind is the nurse who has exceptional skills in IV line insertion. As a new nurse, she may have embraced every opportunity to insert an IV and even volunteered for them. She took extra workshops to improve her skills. You could be an advanced cardiac life support (ACLS) expert and have sought special training to be an instructor.

- What are your talents or natural-born gifts?

Do you have talent in creative thinking? Writing? Are you particularly skilled in presenting data using graphs? Think of your natural talents and include them in your strengths box.

Weaknesses

This is your opportunity to think of areas you need to improve on and things that will potentially put you at a disadvantage in your career.

- What are your negative work habits and traits?

It could be constantly being unprepared when working with a group. Another could be making dominating conversations during meetings. A single occurrence of these may be tolerated, but when these become a habit, it will produce a negative mark on your reputation.

- Does any part of your education or training need improving?

Do you recall your manager recommending a course or a training program for you? Do you find yourself frequently asking a peer to do a specific task for you? Perhaps that's a knowledge or skill gap that can be effectively addressed in a quick workshop.

- What would other people see as your weaknesses?

The Johari window is a self-awareness tool that prompts you to reflect on your personality using four quadrants. One of the quadrants is "unknown to you, known to others." You will be surprised on what others observe in you that you may not be totally aware of.

Opportunities

For an organization or a company, reflecting on opportunities includes looking at new competition or potential areas of growth. See how these apply to your own self-evaluation.

- What is the state of the economy?

Whether the economy is going strong or not gives a good indication of opportunities for promotion, general increase in compensation, or the reverse—possible loss of positions or funding for positions. In some cases, you have to put effort in maintaining your position. Some program-based jobs are funded through grants. When the grant money runs out, the organization can try to figure out a reassignment for you, or you can lose your job completely. One organization received funding for a substance abuse clinic for 5 years. At the end of 5 years, the local government agency that provided funding could no longer sustain the program. The organization attempted to keep the program going for a year and eventually closed the clinic.

- Is your industry growing?

From 2016 to 2026, a 31% growth in overall employment has been projected for nurse anesthetists, nurse midwives, and nurse practitioners (Bureau of Labor Statistics, 2019). For nurse practitioners, some specialties have better opportunities than others. For your field and specialty, do you know how it is growing?

- Is there new technology in your industry?

During our weekly leadership meetings, we are always talking about new mobile applications in providing care, new devices, or new

Table 2.1

Example of SWOT Analysis (Strengths, Weaknesses, Opportunities, and Threats) for the Frontline Clinical Nurse

Strengths	Weaknesses
- Creative (participated in creating screening tool; designed unit visibility board) - Collaborative	- Prioritization - Blood-drawing skills
Opportunities	Threats
- New policy to require specialty certification	- Opening of new ambulatory center, possible transfer

Table 2.2

Example of SWOT Analysis (Strengths, Weaknesses, Opportunities, and Threats) for the Nurse Manager

Strengths	Weaknesses
- Team-building skills - Developed new orientation tools for the unit	- Can get tense in public presentations
Opportunities	Threats
- New functions added to your role	- Diminishing volume in current location

software to use in generating reports. It is easy to feel lost in these conversations if you don't keep yourself up to date. You don't have to learn each system, but at the minimum, be familiar with the ones that you would potentially use in your role.

Threats

Threats include external elements that impact your achievement of your goals.

- Is your industry contracting or changing directions?

This question is prompting you to delve deeper into the opportunities you identified, except that you are looking at it from the perspective of your goals. An example is the movement to encourage nurses to pursue a bachelor's degree. Many organizations are no longer hiring nurses without a BSN degree. How about intensified use of robots in surgery or application of artificial intelligence? Predictive models in artificial intelligence can determine the likelihood that a patient will undergo a specific health event or develop a chronic illness. Nurses will need to learn how to manage these types of information.

Another possible threat is when the industry or your organization opts to getting some jobs outsourced. Still another threat is when the organization stops hiring agency nurses.

■ Is there strong competition for the types of jobs for which you are best suited?

You could be a great fit for the critical care environment, but openings in your local area are limited. Or you have exceptional experience as an educator in nursing informatics, but there is typically just one or two allocated positions for the entire nursing department.

■ What is the biggest external danger to your goals?

Is there a possible merger in your healthcare system that can potentially eliminate some positions? Is there a new policy that would deter you from being qualified to the next level of position?

Reflecting on these questions helps you identify the next steps in your career and set goals, whether short term or long term (Dority, 2017).

Annual Performance Review

To come up with meaningful professional goals, a three-pronged evaluation is expected. A nurse combines reflections from self-evaluation, peer feedback, and manager evaluation to set new goals. In most organizations, this is a mandatory process that occurs annually.

Self-Evaluation

As a first step, review your goals for the past year. Did you accomplish all of them? Do you see any outstanding goal? A basic rule in the appraisal process is that there should be no surprises. This applies to self-evaluation as well. A midyear self-evaluation, whether mandated by your organization or not, is helpful to stay on track. If your organization follows the calendar year timeline for the annual performance review, the midyear evaluation usually happens in June. The domains and items for self-evaluation and manager evaluation are similar. In some cases, you are not required to do a full self-evaluation using a structured form (Table 2.3). Instead, you are asked to write a short narrative that includes a self-reflection on how you performed.

Pointers in Self-Evaluation
■ Include both individual and collaborative accomplishments.
■ Take notes throughout the year or keep a work journal.
■ Demonstrate concrete examples versus writing adjectives.

Table 2.3

Example of Completed Self-Evaluation		
Domain and description	Self-rating (Exceptional, Exceeds expectations, Meets expectations, Does not meet expectations)	Comment
Core Values Upholds and promotes the hospital's core values as demonstrated through patient care and relationship with team members.		
Excellence	Meets expectations	
Compassion	Exceeds expectations	Received two patient letters demonstrating clinical excellence and compassionate care
Respect	Meets expectations	
Autonomy and Accountability	Meets expectations	
Patient Care Management and Care Coordination	Exceeds expectations	Coordinated care for a very complex patient that required placement out of state

Reflective Practice

Alongside self-evaluation, reflective practice contributes to your professional development. In your daily practice, you must constantly evaluate your actions, behaviors, responses, and decisions. It is your professional obligation. Reflective practice helps you to develop coping strategies, enhance interprofessional communication, promote expression of feelings, and make sense of personal emotional practice challenges (Jacobs, 2016).

PEER REVIEW

The American Nurses Association (ANA) defines peer review in nursing as the process by which practicing RNs systematically access, monitor, and make judgments about the quality of nursing care provided by peers as measured against professional standards of practice. Peer review implies that the nursing care delivered by a group of nurses or an individual nurse is evaluated by individuals of the same rank or standing according to established standards of practice.

Why Do Peer Review?

Peer review promotes accountability in practice and promotes healthy communication among peers. It opens an opportunity to provide and receive both positive and constructive feedback on each other's professional practice and development. Leslie, an experienced nurse in interventional radiology, shared her experience in peer review. Her organization implemented a formal peer review process. She selected two peers, with a similar role and rank as her, and sought their feedback.

Leslie received the following feedback:

- Overall, exceeded expectations of both peers
- *Areas of strengths identified:* Great preceptor to new members of the team; unit expert, especially on complex procedures unique to the unit; great involvement in various projects on the unit
- *Areas of opportunity:* Consider applying for clinical advancement; sometimes can be too fast when providing handoff; should try to slow down especially when the incoming nurse is new to the unit

Leslie reflected on these comments and recommendations. She was happy to be regarded as a unit expert. For her, that served as a good validation on how she is regarded on the unit. As for the constructive comments, initially, she was surprised to learn that she had the tendency to give report too swiftly. She sought another colleague's opinion, and the third colleague agreed. Leslie took this to heart and made sure to be more thoughtful and careful moving forward. Leslie incorporated the rest of the feedback received into her goal for the following year.

Benefits of Peer Review

A peer review touches on the same areas covered in an annual performance review, but usually it is much simpler. The following areas are covered: quality of care and service, regard for patient safety and rights, resource utilization, peer-to-peer relationships, contributions to hospital, community, and profession.

Principles of Peer Review (ANA, 1988)

1. *A peer is someone of the same rank.*
   As you saw in Leslie's example, she picked peers of the same rank and role—a clinical nurse to a clinical nurse, nurse educator to another nurse educator, or chief nursing officer (CNO) to another CNO. Someone of the same rank provides an accurate perspective on the expectations of the role, including barriers and challenges encountered in daily practice.

2. *Peer review is practice focused.*

It is not focused on personality or behavior. You are evaluated based on your performance and different aspects of your practice, such as clinical skills and interpersonal communication.

3. *Feedback is timely, routine, and a continuous expectation.*

Although there is a designated time period to do a formal process, feedback should be integrated in the team's routine. In Leslie's case, at the moment when a nursing peer felt rushed during handoff, the feedback should be conveyed as close to the encounter as possible.

4. *Peer review fosters a continuous learning culture of patient safety and best practice.*

Peer review promotes a culture of safety, where everyone feels safe and comfortable in providing and giving feedback. Another common example is skipping critical steps, such as independent double checks, when administering high-alert medications. In a rushed environment, it is easy to just brush aside a missed step like this. When you witness a coworker skipping this step, you should be accountable in providing education or a reminder.

5. *Feedback is not anonymous.*

Without an established relationship, it is challenging to provide in-person feedback. However, to be effective, the process should not be anonymous. This encourages commitment to each other's development and improvement.

6. *Feedback incorporates the nurse's developmental stage.*

Are you new to your area? Are you an experienced leader? The person providing you the feedback should put this into context. In the same way, when you are providing feedback to a peer, make a note of such things.

MANAGER REVIEW

Do you look forward to your annual performance review? Or do you dread it? Take it as a time to have a meaningful conversation with your manager regarding your experience, accomplishments, contributions, and plans.

Think of Your Accomplishments

Did you get certified or finished a degree this year? Did you present at a conference or, perhaps, an event within your organization? If you are in a more advanced or leadership role, did your department accomplish a milestone such as a huge jump in your patient experience score? A colleague who works as a clinical trials research nurse was part of a multicenter study for the first time. This was a very enriching experience for him. It also opened an opportunity for him to showcase the strengths of his organization to other participants in the trial. During his annual performance evaluation, he listed all the projects he completed. Then, he realized he needed to highlight his participation in the multicenter study. This stood out in his manager's review of him and made his manager notice all the other accomplishments he had in a better light. His manager noted his ability to work under tight timelines, follow complex protocols, and being adaptable in his workload.

Reflect on the Past Year's Experience

Overall, was this a great year? What made it great? Or was it more challenging? If your organization just went through a major accreditation process or a regulatory survey, this becomes a part of your experience. I was once part of a team that was moving to a brand-new building. A month prior to the move, two members of our team transitioned and left the organization. This made the move more challenging for the team. Nonetheless, it was very successful. In my annual performance review, I shared my reflection with my manager and noted the resilience and efforts of our team. She acknowledged how I contributed to this major undertaking.

Share Your Contributions

Throughout the year, you are involved in multiple projects that you do not even notice at times. Find time to share this during your annual performance review. Your manager is only one person. Don't assume that she is familiar with every team member's activities and achievements. I interviewed a nurse who has been employed for just over a year and another nurse in a leadership role. See what they shared here.

Newer Nurse
- Drafted a formal reflection on my orientation experience. My preceptor is a member of the Preceptor Committee. With her guidance, I included some suggestions on how to improve the orientation program here on the unit.
- Participated in a survey on how to improve our discharge process.
- Assisted our charge nurse in updating our bulletin board in the break room.

Director of Nursing
- Exceeded targets in turnover and retention rates in four of five units.
- Executive sponsor to three performance improvement projects achieving positive outcomes in patient flow with 8% reduction in lengths of stay, falls reduction of 11%, and catheter-associated urinary tract infections by 23%.
- Launched an organization-wide mentorship program supporting 22 nurses.

Discuss Your Plans

This is a great time to discuss your professional goals. Let your manager know if you are planning to go back to school, aiming for an open position within your department, or intending to expand your experience. Another colleague wanted to go back to school but was concerned about the financial resources required. Her manager just learned about a plan to expand the tuition benefits organization-wide. My colleague would have learned that afterward but was thankful to hear about it directly from her manager. During their conversation, they also discussed how going back to school will impact her work schedule.

Ask Questions

If you feel there are areas of your experience and development that were not discussed, make sure to ask questions. You can ask specific feedback on your performance in areas of opportunity you have identified. You can also share comments received from peers. This open discussion conveys that you are a mature individual and are committed to developing your full potential.

PUTTING IT ALL TOGETHER

You have completed a thorough self-evaluation, sought the feedback of peers, and finished discussing your annual performance review with your manager. What's next? Assimilate comments, ideas, and recommendations received and get ready to set your goals.

Setting Professional Goals

The time-tested format of S-M-A-R-T goals also applies to nursing professional goals. First step, list all your goals and then prioritize. Identify short-term goals from long-term ones.

Here are some examples of goals:

New Nurse
- In the next 12 months, complete continuing education hours to apply for nursing specialty certification.
- In the next 6 months, participate in a project sponsored by our unit council.
- In the next 12 months, complete the nurse residency program and successfully implement my evidence-based practice project.

Midcareer Clinical Nurse
- In the next 6 months, partner with our nurse educator to develop a new learning module in safe patient handling.

- In the next 12 months, mentor and support two nurses toward clinical ladder advancement.

Junior Nursing Faculty
- In the next 2 years, publish a three-part dissertation in peer-reviewed journals.
- In the next 6 months, apply for external funding.

Nurse Practitioner
- In the next 12 months, develop a clinical pathway for patients receiving new hepatitis C treatment.
- In the next 6 months, participate in a performance improvement initiative through the Advanced Practice Nurse Council.

Developing Your CV

A curriculum vitae (CV) is a comprehensive presentation and description of your academic credentials, clinical and academic expertise, and professional accomplishments (Office of Intramural Training and Education, n.d.). Your CV reflects your skills, strengths, and specialties.

Building an Effective and Credible CV

A CV has several main parts: Summary, Personal Information, Education, Professional Experience, Certifications and Licenses, Professional Organizations, Scholarly Presentations, Publications, Awards, and Community Outreach.

Summary

This is an optional section that provides an overview of your credentials, strengths, and objectives.

Personal Information

Here you include basic demographic information: name and contact information.

Education

Starting from the most recent, include school and year of graduation information on your basic nursing education, master's degree, post-master's certificate, and, if any, doctoral and postdoctoral.

Professional Experience

List your current job first, down to your first job. Include place and years of employment, accomplishments, and responsibilities, starting with a verb. Keep it concise. Remember, prospective employers are typically skimming through multiple documents at once and have limited time reviewing each initially. Examples of accomplishments include the following: Co-led a team in catheter-associated urinary tract infection (CAUTI) prevention and achieved 5% reduction within 6 months; achieved $3,500 savings by reducing supply waste brought into patient rooms. Here are examples of responsibilities: Functioned as charge nurse in a 25-bed medical step-down unit in a large academic medical center; served as float nurse in all critical care units in a 500-bed teaching hospital. (See more examples in the sample CV provided in Exhibit 2.1.)

Scholarly Presentations

Add a section on your poster and podium presentations. Specify the title of your presentation, name of conference or meeting, venue, and date. Be consistent in your format. The format provided by the American Psychological Association (APA) as published in the APA manual is widely accepted.

Example:
Jones, A. (2017) CAUTI Reduction in the CCU. *NTI Congress. Boston, MA*

Publications

Start from the most recent, following a chronological order.

Awards

Think of academic awards and excellence-in-service awards.

Community Involvement

This is an important section of your CV and conveys your commitment to serve your community. It also shows your ability to stretch yourself and manage responsibility outside of your normal workload. When I mentor new nurses, I share that when everything else is equal (education, experience, and other accomplishments), the person evaluating you will delve deeper into these categories. In Chapter 4, Being Involved: What's in It for Me?, you will see a more detailed discussion on the benefits and importance of community outreach.

Extramural Activities

This section also reveals your strengths and interests. Here, add your involvement in professional organizations, such as membership or chair position in a committee.

Exhibit 2.1

Example of Completed CV: Advanced Role

Curriculum Vitae

Theresa JXXXX, MSN, RN, NEA-BC
1 Washington Avenue, Town, NJ 01111
311-250-XXXX
theresa_jxxxx@gmail.com

SUMMARY

Innovative nurse leader in diverse clinical settings with excellent track record in building strong team engagement, and clinical and financial outcomes.

PROFESSIONAL EXPERIENCE

Greater New York Medical Center, New York, NY

June 2016-present

Director of Nursing, Oncology Service Line
Provides strategic vision and leadership in the Oncology Service Line in a 700-bed Magnet®-designated academic medical center.

- Established a new bone marrow transplant unit within 6 months of hire
- Increased nurse engagement scores in four domains in all oncology units
- Reduced vacancy rate from 8% to 2% within 9 months

Fox Memorial Medical Center, Another Town, NY
Nurse Manager, Medical Oncology Unit　　**May 2012-June 2016**
Led a team of 56 full time equivalents (FTEs) in an 18-bed medical oncology unit.

- Implemented a new model of interdisciplinary care rounds with demonstrated improvement in three patient experience domains
- Reduced usage of over time by 21% within one year as nurse manager
- Led the development of a new patient acuity tool

Community Hospital of New Jersey, Town, NJ

July 2008-April 2012
Charge Nurse　　July 2010-April 2012
Served as team leader in a 20-bed medical-surgical unit, ensuring the delivery of safe and effective care.

- Supervised assigned clinical nurses in providing direct care to patients

- Developed an electronic self-scheduling system in collaboration with other charge nurses across the hospital

Nurse II, Medical-Surgical Unit   July 2007-June 2010
Provided care for patients in all adult age groups, including assessment and management of the patients in a medical-surgical care setting

EDUCATION

Master of Science in Nursing, National University   **2012**
   Specialty: Nursing Leadership and Administration
Bachelor of Science in Nursing, National University   **2007**

HONORS/SCHOLARSHIPS/AWARDS

Nurse Leader of the Year   **2014**
   Fox Memorial Medical Center
Third Place, Research Poster Category   **June 2010**
   Community Hospital of New Jersey

BOOK CHAPTER PUBLISHED

JXXXX, T. (2018). Preventing infections after bone marrow transplant. In A. Shaw (Ed.). Springer Publishing.

PUBLISHED PEER-REVIEWED ARTICLES

JXXXX, T., & CXXXX, A. (2017). Fall prevention in geriatric patients: Best practices in oncology. *A Journal of Nursing.* https://doi.org/XX.XX.XXXXX

PODIUM & POSTER PRESENTATIONS

JXXXX, T. (2017). Driving nursing engagement: Success stories from nurse leaders. New York Association of Nurse Leaders, Annual Meeting, New York, NY.
JXXXX, T. (2016). Interdisciplinary care rounds: What's next? *Oncology Nursing Congress.* Baltimore, MD.
JXXXX, T. (2015). Collaborative practice in falls prevention. *Oncology Conference.* New York, NY.

PROFESSIONAL SERVICE ACTIVITIES

New York Association of Nurse Leaders
   Member, Professional Practice Panel   July 2016-present
   Reviewer, Poster and Podium Abstracts   2014-2016

CV Versus Résumé

A CV is comprehensive and includes exhaustive information on your background, credentials, and accomplishments. A résumé is a one- to two-page document assembled with a specific objective in mind. It could be for an application of a fellowship, job search, scholarship, or volunteer application. Include relevant information to strengthen your application aligned with your objective. A résumé has the same sections as in a CV, but they are abbreviated.

Exhibit 3.2

Example of Résumé: Frontline Clinical Nurse Position

RÉSUMÉ

Theresa JXXXX, MSN, RN, NEA-BC
1 Washington Avenue, Town, NJ 01111
311-250-XXXX
theresa_jxxxx@gmail.com

SUMMARY

Experienced critical care nurse with demonstrated excellence in clinical decision-making skills and evidence-based practice. Interested in a senior clinical nurse position in a teaching hospital.

PROFESSIONAL EXPERIENCE

Greater New York Medical Center, New York, NY
June 16-present
Clinical Nurse III, Surgical Intensive Care Unit (SICU)
Served as team leader in a 15-bed SICU, ensuring the delivery of safe and effective care.

Fox Memorial Medical Center, Another Town, NY
Clinical Nurse I   **May 2012-June 2016**
Provided care for patients in all adult age groups, including assessment and management of the patients in a medical-surgical care setting.

EDUCATION

Master of Science in Nursing, National University   **2013**
Bachelor of Science in Nursing, National University   **2007**

LICENSES AND CERTIFICATIONS

New York   **Expiration: Dec 2019**

HONORS/SCHOLARSHIPS/AWARDS

Employee of the Year   June 2014
Fox Memorial Medical Center

POSTER PRESENTATION

JXXXX, T. (2017). Making bedside handoff work for your unit. *Annual EBP/Research Symposium.* Fox Memorial Medical Center, White Plains, NY.

PROFESSIONAL SERVICE ACTIVITIES

SICU Unit Council
Member   July 2015-2017

Identifying Gaps in Your CV

Use your CV as a tool to identify gaps in your professional growth and development. You may have presented regularly in local and national conferences but have no experience in publication. You may have multiple certifications but have not really thought about going back to school. There is no right or wrong answer. Go back to what goals you have set for yourself, including your timelines.

Developing Your Professional E-Portfolio

A professional e-portfolio or web-based portfolio is an electronic repository of credentials, professional work, and other documents relevant to your professional career. It is an alternative to storing your documents in a physical binder or a box. With an e-portfolio, you can share your documents and work with someone in your professional network remotely. It is likened to an electronic version of your CV plus the ability to electronically attach related work. You can attach copies of published articles and scholarly presentations. You can enhance it with graphics and include links about your professional accomplishments (https://eportfolioreview.wordpress.com/eportfolio-list).

Parts of a Professional E-Portfolio

You can select from many templates or formats for your e-portfolio offered by various e-portfolio systems. In general, you have a home page, and then you can create categories or tabs. Within each category, you build the content and present your professional background and accomplishments through brief narratives and bullet points. Be creative!

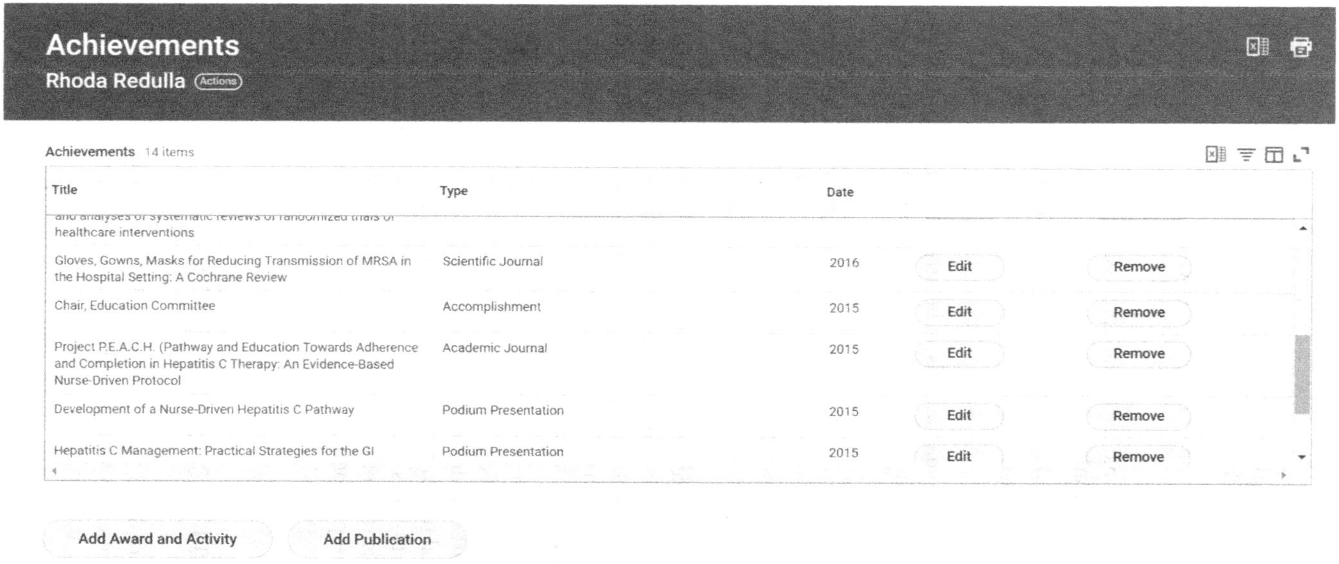

Figure 2.1 Snapshot of a professional e-portfolio.

Home Page

This is the first page that viewers see when they open your portfolio. Add your professional headshot and a brief introduction. Make this page warm and inviting.

Optional attachment: Short introductory video or a voice recording.

Background

Present your educational credentials, professional experience, licenses, and specialty certifications.

Recommended attachment: CV or résumé, copy of nursing license, copy of specialty certification.

Accomplishments

Here you showcase your awards, scholarly presentations, publications, involvement in professional organizations, and community outreach.

Recommended attachments: Award certificates, copies of peer-reviewed articles, a weblink to show involvement in professional organizations, photos, link to blog.

Other Sections

You can add any additional sections you would like to highlight. If you are involved in global health, you can share that work here. A nurse who has obtained a fellowship may want to present these activities here. Others also add a section on reflection or journal entries on their professional experiences.

Recommended attachments: Photos, relevant documents to showcase your interests and work.

Within the last decade, nursing schools have used the e-portfolio as an educational tool to facilitate reflective learning. Nursing students use the e-portfolio as a repository of reflections and journal entries during practicum. Some master's or doctoral degrees also integrate the use of an e-portfolio in the curriculum. My current organization included the e-portfolio to our employee human resources management system.

CREATING YOUR PROFESSIONAL ROAD MAP

You have completed your self-evaluation, sought the feedback of peers, and reviewed your annual performance with your manager. You have also updated your CV and reflected on the gaps you identified. You are ready to create your professional road map. First, draft your goals and then write strategies to get there that you can commit to.

Long-Term Goals

A long-term goal is one that requires 3 to 5 years to complete.
Goal: Become a certified nurse practitioner in 3 years.

Strategies

- Attend an information session. Learn about the admission requirements. Meet current faculty and students to obtain more insights on the program.
- Submit your official transcripts for evaluation. The admission officer can provide advice if you are able to enroll in the program without any prerequisite courses. If you are an international student or a graduate of a foreign nursing program, you will need to have your credentials evaluated by an approved credentials evaluation agency.
- Submit admission requirements. Check for any required tests, such as the Graduate Record Examination (GRE).
- Check the financial requirements. Many organizations have a tuition assistance or reimbursement program. Obtain more information about this through your human resources office. You may also need to inquire about other financing options, such as securing a student loan. The school can provide more information on these resources, too.

Short-Term Goals

A short-term goal is one that requires 6 to 12 months to complete. Goal: Apply for promotion through the clinical ladder advancement program.

Strategies

- Discuss your goal with your manager. Obtain more information on the program.
- Request an application packet. Even if you do not meet all the requirements immediately, this will help you prepare for any missing elements.
- Seek a mentor. Reach out to someone who has successfully obtained a clinical ladder promotion.
- Identify gaps in your application. If the application requires that you are involved in a unit or hospital initiative, work with your manager. You can also partner with another peer who has a similar goal as you.

Resources in Professional Advancement

Take advantage of available professional development programs in your organization or those offered by external agencies. Examples include fellowship or mentoring programs. These are open for application typically with limited slots. You are assigned a mentor and afforded paid time to do your project. Sometimes you also receive extra financial support to implement your project.

A fellowship or mentoring program usually runs for 1 year with a formal development plan or curriculum. (See Table 2.4 for an example of a nursing fellows development plan.)

SAMPLE PROGRAM

Nursing Excellence Fellowship, National Hemophilia Foundation

Eligibility

The purpose of the National Hemophilia Foundation Nursing Fellowship is to provide support for a registered nurse currently employed or interested in hemophilia care to conduct nursing research or clinical projects.

- Endorsement by a federally funded hemophilia treatment center is recommended.
- Only registered nurses from an accredited nursing school enrolled in a graduate nursing program or practicing hemophilia nursing care may apply.
- Collaboration with multidisciplinary care providers and/ or between two or more hemophilia centers is accepted and encouraged. Collaboration efforts may include, for example, social work, physical therapy, and genetics. It thus may be possible for a hemophilia center team to apply jointly for two or more of the nursing, social work, and physical therapy excellence fellowships as a cooperative project or research endeavor. Additionally, regional applications will be considered.

Funding

Each year one new research fellowship of up to $13,500 will be awarded.

Leadership Education Programs

Many organizations offer either in-person or online leadership programs. Topics range from time management to team building and communication. Your human resources talent development department organizes these programs. For online education, you may already have this on your online learning management portal.

Table 2.4

12-Month Nursing Fellows Development Plan (2019)

The goal of the 12-month development plan is to support nursing fellows in their current roles and facilitate professional growth and development. Fellows and mentors meet to discuss and develop an individualized plan for each fellow.

Development Focus	Development focus captures the specific skills, abilities, or experiences you need to prepare for current and future success. This area of focus may reflect a specific competency or technical skill. Examples include: - Enhance oral presentation skills. - Broaden my organizational perspective by leading and contributing to projects outside my areas of expertise.
Exposure	Exposure means experiences with new people, ideas, technology, processes, and practices. This may include: - Strategic involvement in a committee - Involvement in a professional organization - Shadowing a role
Education	What education needs should be addressed? - Degree program - Professional certification - Leadership program
Risks/ Barriers	This may include other work-related competing priorities and nursing fellow–specific circumstances and behaviors.

Source: Modified with permission from BJC Healthcare Leadership Competencies Program.

SUCCESS STORY

Kathy A. Baker, PhD, APRN, ACNS-BC, FAAN

Associate Professor
Director, Nursing Research and Scholarship
Deputy Director, Center for Translational Research: A JBI Center of Excellence
Texas Christian University
Harris College of Nursing and Health Sciences;
Editor-in-Chief, *Gastroenterology Nursing*

Describe your professional nursing journey (include highlights of your career).

I really didn't know what I was getting myself into when I chose nursing as an undergraduate student. I really wanted to be a teacher but felt I was being directed (from a spiritual perspective) into nursing. There was a couple who were close family friends that pushed me to look at nursing. She was a nurse, and he was a hospital administrator. After a great deal of thinking and praying, I ended up declaring nursing as my major and have never looked back! I was always a good student, but I had to work hard to be successful. And nursing school was more difficult than I had expected. I had to really work at understanding such a broad body of knowledge. Then connecting that broad knowledge base to patient decision-making was even more overwhelming. But I loved it and had great mentors along the way that helped me push through. As a student, that family friend who was a hospital administrator facilitated my working as a patient aide while I was in my junior and senior years of nursing school. That experience really contributed a lot to my understanding of patient care from doctor's orders, to pharmacology, procedures, "typical" care plans, and healthcare team relationships. I felt very comfortable in the acute care world because of that opportunity when I finally entered nursing practice as a new graduate.

After graduating with my BSN, I was accepted into one of the "early" nurse residencies. I worked in a step-down unit with ventilated patients for a few weeks and then, after much insistence, was allowed to work as a new graduate in a surgical intensive care unit. This was not typical at that point in time. Thankfully, I was naive enough to not recognize that my success or failure would open or close doors for other new graduates! Thankfully, that experience was positive and after a few years in SICU, I moved to MICU where I took my first leadership position as evening unit manager. A nurse colleague was pursuing her masters in nursing while I was working in SICU and encouraged me to take an advanced pathology course at her university to prepare to take the certified critical care registered nurse (CCRN) examination. Naive as I was, I found out I had to apply to graduate school to take the course, so I did. And because I finally understood what I was learning and could immediately apply that knowledge to my patients, I kept going, eventually obtaining a master's degree with a dual focus as a clinical nurse specialist and nurse administrator.

In the MICU, we often scoped patients at the bedside and that is where I fell in love with endoscopy. The gastroenterologists were great teachers and very patient to answer all of my questions about what I was seeing. They connected my endoscopy experience to implications for the patient's care and I was enthralled. From MICU, I actually became the hospital-wide house supervisor for evening shift and learned a great deal about crisis intervention and problem-solving. Next, I became head nurse of a well mom-baby unit that also cared for high-risk antepartum patients. I was asked to apply for that role because the nursing administrators wanted someone who enjoyed teaching and supporting staff to help the nurses expand their focus from just paying attention to postpartum care to whole-patient care. It was a great experience.

My love for endoscopy never left me, and when an opportunity came for me to apply to be the GI Nurse Manager at the county teaching hospital across the street, I jumped at the chance. I was delighted to be selected and worked with amazing nurse colleagues, GI fellows, and GI attending physicians. I loved the teaching environment and the challenges of working in that setting. While there, we doubled the size of our unit, so I was very involved in designing, purchasing, and opening the new GI unit. My love for research and teaching was supported while I was in this role, and eventually, I pursued an academic career that allowed me to bring undergraduate students back to my former hospital. I loved the familiarity of taking undergraduate students into such a positive learning environment and always found a way to have my students experience at least one observational day in the GI procedure area!

Shortly before I left clinical practice to enter academia, I was solicited to apply for the editor of *Gastroenterology Nursing*. Obtaining that position has been a highlight of my nursing career as it has allowed me to stay connected to GI nursing practice, opened doors for me to meet and share with colleagues around the world, and gave me an outlet for the reading and writing that I enjoy. A few years into academia, I went on to pursue my PhD in nursing and now work with graduate nursing students pursuing their master's or doctorate in nursing.

From the perspective of creating your professional road map: What would you advice nurses who are just starting on their nursing careers? Nurses who are midcareer?

I was quite naive about career development as a nurse. My dream job as a new graduate was to land a job in intensive care, but as I previously noted, new graduates were not yet allowed to enter ICU until they had had a couple of years of general nursing experience. It did not take me long to see that there are certain personality types drawn to the different specialties in nursing. I found this fascinating and very telling. For nurses just starting their careers, I would encourage them to pursue their passion, but be flexible. The diversity of my career has allowed me to develop a broad foundation for my career. None of the opportunities, including graduate school, were part of my vision for how my career would unfold. I really thought I would be happy being an ICU nurse for my entire nursing career. Yet, I was craving new opportunities for learning and growing just 2 short years after graduating and landing that dream job in ICU. As doors opened along my journey, I pursued different experiences, and all of them have been valuable to me as I progressed in my career.

For nurses who are midcareer, I would encourage you to follow your heart. If you love what you do, don't feel pressure to pursue something else. You may be right where you need to be! But you might consider exploring a new nursing role in your same setting or stepping up into informal leadership positions like serving on a committee in your practice setting or taking a leadership role in your professional organization. And if you do feel an urge for a change, don't be afraid to pursue a new specialty or a new role. Every job I pursued in nursing always seemed to build upon previous experiences, making my practice (and my life) much fuller because of the diversity in roles and settings I experienced.

What are you most proud of?

I am most proud of being inducted as a fellow in the American Academy of Nursing. The recognition by my peers that I have made a sustained contribution to nursing that is worthy of recognition in very humbling and rewarding.

What is your aspiration for the nursing profession?

My aspiration for nursing is that our contributions are fully recognized and valued by society. I find most people do not understand the rigor involved in pursuing a nursing degree, the level of responsibility we have in the healthcare arena, and the influence we hold in advocating for what is best for a patient and their family. I want nurses to practice to their full scope as an equitable member of the healthcare team and to be valued as a critical leader in society.

Your commitment to professional development?

When does professional development end? During one of my graduate classes, a classmate who was about 2 years from retirement was thinking out loud. We were reviewing an upcoming assignment that involved reading several chapters of our textbook and writing a big paper. She said it was times like that when she wonders why she decided to make life complicated. If she was not in school, she could be just relaxing in the evenings or enjoying her weekends. But she was quick to respond. She confessed that it was a tough decision to go back to school. What would she do with her degree? She was definitely not looking forward to a promotion at that point in her career. It was a gift she wanted to do for herself. She said that, all her life, she was wondering what she could have accomplished had she decided to go back to school sooner.

As healthcare professionals, you are individually responsible for planning and carrying out continuing professional development activities, ensuring your relevance to current practice and career development (Brekelmans, Maassen, Poell, Westrate, & Geurdes, 2016). Your organization may provide resources or facilitate access to professional development and programs, but you are ultimately accountable for your advancement.

Key Points

- In setting professional goals, commit to doing periodic self-evaluations, seeking feedback from peers, and reflecting on your manager's evaluation.
- Maintain an up-to-date CV and invest time in developing your professional e-portfolio.
- Pursue diverse experiences and training opportunities. Possibilities in creating your professional road map are endless.

References

American Nurses Association (1988). *Peer review guidelines*. Kansas City, MO: Author.

Brekelmans, G., Maassen, S., Poell, R. F., Weststrate, J., & Geurdes, E. (2016). Factors influencing nurse participation in continuing professional development activities: Survey results from the Netherlands. *Nurse Education Today, 40*, 13–19. doi:10.1016/j.nedt.2016.01.028

Bureau of Labor Statistics. (2019). *Nurse anesthetists, nurse midwives, and nurse practitioners*. Retrieved from https://www.bls.gov/ooh/healthcare/nurse-anesthetists-nurse-midwives-and-nurse-practitioners.htm

Dority. (2017). *Career check-up with Dr. Elaine Foster: Part 1*. https://www.americansentinel.edu/blog/2017/08/18/use-a-swot-analysis-to-build-your-nursing-or-healthcare-career/

Hickey, K. (2018). Developing and sustaining a career as a transdisciplinary nurse scientist. *Journal of Nursing Scholarship, 50*(1), 20–27. doi:10.1111/jnu.12359

Jacobs, S. (2016). Reflective learning, reflective practice. *Nursing, 46*(5), 62–64. doi:10.1097/01.NURSE.0000482278.79660.f2

Martin, M. (2015). *How to do a personal SWOT analysis*. Retrieved from https://www.businessnewsdaily.com/5543-personal-swot-analysis.html

Office on Intramural Training and Education. (n.d.). *Hints for writing your resume/CV*. Retrieved from https://www.training.nih.gov/writing_your_resume

Embracing Opportunity

Rhoda R. Redulla

"It's easy to be at a place where you know what you're doing and are the nurse consultant or deputy to the chief nurse. But being at the top of your game can be a little stifling if you don't push boundaries and seek external opportunities. Go into the unknown."

—Joanne Bosanquet, MBE, RN

A former mentor loved to share this fable on opportunity whenever he speaks on strategic planning and professional development. This is a conversation between a traveler and a statue of "opportunity."

Traveler: *Say, if the cause you may reveal, why thus supported on a wheel?*
Opportunity: *The wheel my rapid course implies, Like that with constant speed flies.*
Traveler: *Wings on your feet?*
Opportunity: *I'm prone to soar, neglected, I return no more.*
Traveler: *But why behind depriv'd of hair?*
Opportunity: *Escaped, that none may seize me there.*
Traveler: *Your locks unbound conceal your eyes?*
Opportunity: *Because, I chiefly court disguise.*

The key takeaway of this story is not to overlook opportunity. When opportunity comes, and if it is aligned with your personal and professional goals, be prepared to seize it.

Sometimes, you don't even notice how great it is. As the statue said, "I chiefly court disguise."

In this chapter, you will learn about how to move forward when a promising opportunity comes your way. This could be a new role, promotion, or new organization. It will feature examples of how nurses succeeded simply by being at the right place at the right time, and being prepared for it.

The last part of the chapter also includes strategies on how to manage opportunities that do not work out as you have planned.

CHANGE IN ROLE: WHAT'S NEXT?

You have been in an advanced clinical role for several years now. You are really comfortable in your department and are the go-to person for almost everyone on your unit. You have been a preceptor to many nurses, and some of them have transitioned to other roles. You are near completion of your master's degree. You have been involved in multiple initiatives. What's next? Another scenario: You have been a program director in an undergraduate nursing program for over 5 years now. You are involved in university-wide projects and quite content with how your program has evolved. What's next?

At your recent performance appraisal, your manager asked you about your future goals. You were not fully prepared to answer this question. Your manager mentioned about several positions that present an opportunity for you to advance in your career. Not that the department would want to lose you but your manager planted this seed in your head to start thinking about the next steps in your career.

Here are other roles that can be a stepping-stone for anyone who is considering advancing their nursing career or transitioning to a leadership role.

- Nurse coordinator
- Nurse educator
- Nursing project manager
- Clinical nurse specialist
- Nursing supervisor

For current nurse leaders, depending on your area of specialization, the following roles may be the next steps for you:

- Assistant vice-president
- Chief nursing officer (CNO)
- School of nursing dean
- Director of nursing (DON)

EMBRACING AN OPPORTUNITY FOR PROMOTION

Getting a promotion may not be something within your full control, but you can definitely initiate or influence it. Paige (2015) shared some advice to get closer to your goal of being promoted.

- Don't wait to get started.
- Be a team player.
- Find a mentor.
- Follow your passion.
- Go back to school.
- Read voraciously.
- Volunteer for assignments.
- Don't let ambition get out of control.
- Use your organization's career ladder.

Nurses are promoted in several pathways: promotion from general to specialty area, promotion to an advanced practice role, promotion to a nursing management position, promotion to a nonnursing management position, or promotion to a senior leadership position. In academia, promotion involves advancing into tenured status. In the hospital setting, another mechanism for promotion is the clinical ladder program.

Clinical Ladder Program

The clinical ladder is a structured system to provide career advancement to direct care nurses while they remain in the clinical setting (Loyola University Health System, 2013). In one organization, the following set of criteria encompasses their clinical ladder program. The same set of criteria is typical in many organizations (Kalwacki, Fellman, & Torosian, 2015).

- Meet or exceed all expectations on their annual performance evaluation and obtain their director's signature to validate their eligibility for recognition.
- Submit an application packet consisting of their Professional Development Activity Points List and a portfolio of supporting documentation.
- Submit a clinical exemplar reflecting on a clinical experience that demonstrates exemplary professional practice (first-time applicants only).

The levels of advancement most often reflect Patricia Benner's Novice to Expert Model. Table 3.1 is an example of the different levels from Hackensack University Medical Center.

Table 3.1

Clinical Ladder Levels (Novice to Expert Model)	
Level I	Entry level, focused primarily on developing basic knowledge and skills.
Level II	Competent staff nurse focused on expanding knowledge and skills, capable of daily charge role. Assumes an increasing level of leadership, while seeking mentorship.
Level III	Experienced and highly skilled staff nurse, clinically proficient and recognized for knowledge and skills by peers. Has an emerging leadership style and functions consistently and autonomously in this role.
Level IV	Possesses clinical expertise within a defined specialty. Demonstrates performance improvement, research process, evidence-based practice, and peer mentoring.

Source: From Hackensack University Medical Center. (2019). *Designed to recognize and motivate ongoing development of expertise and professionalism of our nurses.* Retrieved from https://www.hackensackumc.org/nursing/professional -development/clinical-ladders/

Some organizations have levels up to five or six, providing more opportunities for nurses to advance. Degrees higher than a BSN may be required, or at least enrollment in a master's program, for Level IV and higher.

In a study that looked into the skills required in nurses' career advancement, Sheikhib, Fallahi-Khoshnab, Mohammadi, and Oskouie reported three themes with subthemes that emerged (2016):

- Interpersonal capabilities (interaction: ladder to progression, sensitivity to hospital problems, being a good mentor, sensitivity to hospital issues)
- Career competency for success (experimenting: key to career progression, management ability, clinical skills mastery)
- Personal capacities (attachment of importance to work, commitment to professional values)

The findings of the study affirmed that personal, interpersonal, and functional skills can facilitate nurses' career advancement. You will also notice that one key element to advancement is "experimenting," which involves taking calculated risks or leaving your comfort zone. Raso (2013, p. 6) honed in on leaving her comfort zone and shared her personal experience and reflection. "I've personally made agonizing decisions to leave wonderful organizations to take on new challenges. In fact, you may have noticed that my byline is a new role for me after more than 10 years as CNO of a wonderful organization where, yes, I was comfortable. It takes strength and some moxie to make this leap. I've also responded to gentle 'pushes' by my mentors to take on different ventures or volunteer roles. These decisions have always proven to be wise. Remember, even failures are golden opportunities for learning and growth."

Promotion From General to Specialty Area

Although it is no longer surprising to see nurses starting in specialized clinical areas right after graduation, many nurses start their careers on a general floor. After obtaining 1 to 2 years of experience, nurses start exploring options to work in a specialized unit such as the surgical intensive care unit, operating room, or cardiac catheterization department.

Pointers for Transition

- Before accepting the new position, inquire about existing transition or gateway to specialty programs. Sometimes hospitals also have specialty-specific nurse residency programs that include experienced nurses.
- Have an open discussion with your manager on the duration of your orientation in the specialty area.
- Ask about a self-assessment tool of your experience and skills. This will help them match you with the right preceptor. If there is no tool, convey your strengths and developing skills.

Promotion to an Advanced Practice Role

Nurse Practitioner Role Transition

Challenges in transition to practice can be experienced across many areas of nursing, including by advanced practice registered nurses (APRNs). For instance, nurse practitioners (NPs) are entering specialized areas of practice immediately after graduation from NP education and certification and find themselves employed in specialized areas such as oncology. Swiftly shifting to and achieving a knowledge base in this highly specialized area of medicine coupled with the stress of the new NP role can lead to a very difficult orientation and transition period (Hoffman, Klein, & Rosenzweig, 2017). NP turnover is twice that of physicians (Bureau of Labor Statistics, 2016). It could be worse in certain specialties than others. Currently, there is a critical shortage of neonatal NPs in the United States (Moss & Jackson, 2019). There is a strong imperative to support the transition and retention of NPs.

- Review the plan for your orientation. A structured and formal orientation process is one of the key factors to your successful transition (Barnes, 2015).
- Find an experienced and motivated mentor or apply for a mentorship program.

Promotion to a Nursing Management Position

Nurses who become nurse managers may receive little or no training or support during the transition process (Pilat & Miriam, 2019). Vacancy in a management position creates opportunities for nurses in direct care to move up to a management role (Doria, 2015). Some may be more prepared than others. Most new managers may not even know the expectations of the role or competencies that they need to have. One study described the transition of certified registered nurse anesthetists (CRNAs) to the manager role. The findings showed that many managers did not seek management opportunities but fell into their management role without management experience. During this critical transition, how can the new nurse manager be successful (Martens, Motz, & Stump, 2018)?

Pointers for Transition

- Complete a self-assessment using a formal competency checklist. The American Organization for Nursing Leadership (AONL, 2015) has developed one.
- Seek out a good mentor. Minsky and Peter (2019) described a "trusted mentor" as someone who has made difficult decisions, taken risks and managed those risks, and who has the self-awareness to give good counsel.
- Ask to be considered for a leadership development program.
- Inquire about available courses, instructor-led or on-demand through online access, based on your identified needs.
- Clarify expectations. In some cases, such as CRNAs and NPs, APRNs may still be required to fulfill their clinical roles, which are already challenging enough.

The Nurse Manager Competencies

The AONL developed nurse manager competencies. They are a useful guide for both aspiring and current nurse managers. For senior nurse leaders, they are helpful in supporting the development of nurse managers and succession planning. The AONL Nurse Manager Competencies are comprised of three domains: the Science (Managing the Business); the Leader Within (Creating the Leader in Yourself); and the Art (Leading the People). Descriptions of each domain are available at https://www.aonl.org/system/files/media/file/2019/06/nurse-manager-competencies.pdf.

Promotion From Mid- to Upper-Level Management

The transition from mid- to upper-level management can vary, and it is driven by the type of role involved. The process may be easier when the transition occurs within the same organization or within the same discipline or specialty. One could be a DON for oncology, moving up to a vice-president for a cancer center. Another could be a DON for the perioperative services, moving up as a CNO or vice-president for operations. These scenarios can translate into different experiences in transitioning to the role. Regardless, there are common strategies or advice to keep in mind. The Forbes Coach Council (2016) shared the "12 Pitfalls When Moving From Mid- to Upper-Level Management." Here, you will see some of them with highlights of the comments for each.

- Changing Focus
  - Be sure to adjust the bigger view in your new role.
- Shifting From the "Doer" Mentality
  - Do not be trapped with ineffective delegation.
- Assumptions
  - Clarify expectations of the role and ask questions during your transition.
- Moving From Problem-Solving to Opportunity Seeking
  - Senior-level managers are expected to spark inspiration, innovation, and strategic agility.
- Lacking "Lead-by-Example" Attitude.
  - You have a strong impact when you "lead by example" because of the larger effect you have on your subordinates.
- Rethinking and Redefining Relationships
- Developing Strategic Thinking
  - The skills aligned with strategic thinking are trust, self-awareness, relating, accountability, focus, empathy, decisiveness, resilience, courage, systems thinking, and vision.

EMBRACING AN OPPORTUNITY OF ROLE EXPANSION

In healthcare, changes can happen frequently or unexpectedly. In the clinical arena, you are expected to be prepared for these changes all the time. How about when the change involves the scope of your role?

A colleague was quite happy leading a general pediatric unit. She had just successfully launched an interdisciplinary rounds initiative which led to some quick wins in patient experience and improvement in quality. In partnership with the nursing professional development specialist, her unit just reviewed and revised their annual competencies. They are now gearing up for the annual competency validation. The hospital was within The Joint Commission regulatory survey window. My colleague was also intensely preparing her team on the top 10 compliance checklist that was just released. She was very comfortable and confident in her role. One morning, she was asked to meet with her immediate supervisor, the DON and the CNO. At the meeting, the DON, who also has oversight of the newborn nursery, and CNO asked that she take on the newborn nursery as an additional unit. The current nurse manager will be leaving. Should she accept this opportunity? Or is this more of a mandate for her to take on? What can she do to ensure that she will be successful in this expanded role?

In a survey by Zastocki (2010), themes of what nurse managers want to increase their job satisfaction were identified. The same framework can be used when requesting support in an expanded role.

a. **Work–life Balance**

Themes mainly revolved around scheduling (flexible scheduling, more time-off). When you are asked to take on an expanded role, be open about your concerns on scheduling. If this added responsibility means you will be working longer hours, are you able to leave earlier on days when it is not too busy? The goal is to avoid putting you in a situation vulnerable to burnout.

b. **Support**

Do you currently have clerical support? If you do, will the current person be helping you in this additional role. If not, what existing responsibilities do you have that can be reassigned or eliminated altogether? Are you supporting a committee that entails significant follow-up work after each meeting?

c. **Acknowledgment**

In the survey, the themes were recognition of the difficulty of the role, accountability from other departments, and respect from the CNO/nursing director. When you are given an expanded responsibility, you assume that everyone is aware of this. However, make sure that this communication occurs to all parties involved.

d. **Compensation**

This is important. Salary should be commensurate with job responsibilities. You can also look at other existing benefits and see how you can maximize them to your advantage.

e. Leadership/Professionalism

What professional development support can you tap into as your leadership role expands?

f. Autonomy

When discussing autonomy, "no micromanaging" comes up. This is relevant and can make or break an employee's engagement or chances to succeed. However, the essence of your autonomy as a leader is best reflected in your ability to make needed change.

As a leader, changes in your scope of leadership may mean being moved to a different department or unit. A nurse manager in a medical-surgical unit could be asked to be moved to a specialty unit. A vacancy in a DON position typically requires another DON to cover the vacant role until it is filled. On occasion, due to financial constraints, the role change can become permanent. An effective and resilient leader is agile and is prepared for these changes. When the prospective changes seem to be overwhelming, do not hesitate to seek advice and speak up.

Embracing Opportunity in a New Organization

Wiggins (2017) offered sage advice on how to set yourself up for success in a new organization. New faces and names, new structures, policies and procedures. How do you successfully plot a route through all of this "new"? The focus of the article was on the transition of managers but can easily be translated into other roles.

- Go on a listening tour for key information to help you to be successful. Hear stories from your colleagues. Ask about their current projects. I am a huge believer on the value of shadowing.
- Learn about organizational culture. How are employees dressed? What acronyms are used?
- Outline team expectations. Be cognizant of how your new team feels about having you as their new leader. Some members may be mourning the loss of the previous leadership. Meet with each of your direct reports one-on-one.
  - Tell each of them what's important to you; this begins the framework for the work you'll do together.
  - Ask what they aspire to do in their careers and keep notes to help them achieve their goals.
  - Ask what are the most important things you can do to help them improve their ability to meet their goals.
- Interview your supervisor.

- Get access. This is huge—access to the computer system, being added to email distribution lists, physical access to restricted areas, and so on.

Crossroads: Feeling Stalled and Confused

Throughout this chapter, I have been urging you to be prepared and embrace new opportunities. In reality, there are many times in your career when you might feel undervalued, unaccomplished, or unsure of where to take your career. I sometimes find myself lost in thought, thinking "Do I see myself doing the same things in the next year or two?" I feel I have accomplished much in the last few years and feel quite content professionally. But how long will that feeling last?

As you gain experience and skills, expect to have more complex responsibilities tied to enhancing the organization's revenue. You are expected to create and drive purposeful change. Aside from seeking a mentor, Minsky and Peter (2019) invite you to ask yourself the following questions when feeling stalled or when in what they call a midcareer rut. I've transformed them into a reflection and action plan box for you (Exhibit 3.1).

Exhibit 3.1

Reflection and Action Plan Questionnaire

Ask Yourself	YES: Proceed to next column NO: No further action required	What step can you do in the next week to address this?	What step can you do in the next month to address this?
Do you spend each day getting through what's on your calendar and to-do list without asking yourself if your involvement makes a difference?	Yes: Proceed to next column	Review my calendar and identify appointments and meetings that do not contribute to my individual priorities this year.	Identify strategies on how my involvement and contributions can make a difference to my individual development plan or organizational goals.
Are you critical of change without truly considering the likely consequences of maintaining the status quo or the potential rewards of change?			

(continued)

Exhibit 3.1

Reflection and Action Plan Questionnaire (*continued*)

Ask Yourself	YES: Proceed to next column NO: No further action required	What step can you do in the next week to address this?	What step can you do in the next month to address this?
Do you avoid or procrastinate making decisions that you perceive as creating more work for you or as taking on risk you would like to avoid?			
Are you seeking help to understand how the work of leading is different from the work of managing?			
Have you articulated what kind of leader you are and what kind of leader you want to become?			

Relocating for a New Job: How Do You Do It?

You accepted a new job that requires you to relocate. Moving to a new job can be stressful enough; then add the complexity of moving to a new city on top of that. Moving with your family, especially little kids, becomes exponentially challenging. Moving for work involves adjustment both personally and professionally. Aside from adjusting to new coworkers and new organizational culture, add new commute, new home, new school for your kids, and a range of other new changes and challenges (Evans, 2019).

Pointers for Transition

- Keep your life simple. Avoid overloading your schedule. Focus on the basics first.
- Stick to your familiar routine (e.g., packing lunches the night before, early morning walk on the weekends).
- Find your personal and professional network. Ask for recommendations at work for places and clubs aligned with your interests. In my town, we have a "Newcomers' Club" that helps individuals and families transition during their first year (Evans, 2019).

Reaching Your Full Potential

Once in a higher or formal leadership role, maximizing your full potential may not be top on your agenda. You can get caught up fulfilling the needs of your department and accomplishing your current goals but fail to think of your own development as a leader. Organizations have leader development programs, and you are encouraged to take advantage of these opportunities. However, there could be limited slots available at one time. Without a formal program open, it is good to think about aspects of your development that you can work on. The Center for Creative Leadership (2019) has established a program for leaders to develop the following skills:

- Developing self-awareness
- Giving and receiving feedback
- Performance conversations
- Active listening
- Coaching and developing others
- Influencing with and without authority
- Learning agility

Both through formal and informal means, be deliberate in seeking experiences and support to develop in these areas. With the ever-changing terrain in healthcare, you may find yourself in unexpected positions to decide about changing scopes and roles. Most of the time, you need to make a decision swiftly.

PUTTING IT ALL TOGETHER

Many times in your career, you will see yourself finding new opportunities, sometimes at the most unexpected time in your life. Other times, the perfect opportunity seems to find you when you feel you are not prepared. Other times, you catch yourself being restless, not able to decide if you are happy about your career or ready to move on to the next chapter. What is your ultimate career goal? What makes you thrive? What excites you? Guided by your north star, review your professional and personal calendar for the coming month and consider which interactions bring you closer to your objectives and which pull you further away. Are you collaborating with people who share your values or who can teach you new ways of looking at things? Do you thrive when interacting with people who are upbeat, analytical, calm, or ambitious (Cross, 2019)?

SUCCESS STORY

Joanne Bosanquet, MBE, RN

Chief Executive Officer, Foundation of Nursing Studies (FoNS), London, England

Describe your professional nursing journey, including your current role.

In 2019, I took a big leap in my career and assumed the role as chief executive for the FoNS (Foundation of Nursing Science). It is a nonprofit organization, committed to working with nurses and healthcare and social work teams to develop and share innovative ways of improving practice and embedding person-centered cultures of care. Prior to this role, I worked both at the front line and in public health, nursing, and health visiting, and I also worked with the Royal College of Nursing. I am a Queen's Nurse, a fellow of the Queen's Nursing Institute, and a visiting professor at the University of Surrey. I also lecture across the United Kingdom and was awarded an honorary doctorate by Greenwich University in 2017.

One of the highlights of my career was being nominated for an honor as MBE (Member of the Order of the British Empire) for services to health and nursing in 2013. My MBE was awarded by Her Majesty The Queen at Windsor Castle following a phenomenal experience working on pandemic flu in 2009 and as part of the London Olympics Health Protection Team in 2012. Later that year, I was appointed as the first deputy chief nurse for Public Health England and spent the next 5-1/2 years developing this role and creating strategic networks and stakeholder relationships across the system, and internationally.

What are one or two pieces of advice that you can share for new nurses as they create their professional road maps? How can nurses reach their full potential?

My personal mantra is "We are global nurses," or #WeAreGlobal Nurses. We have responsibility globally and to each other. My advice is that regardless of your role, you have the ethical and moral responsibility to utilize your position in the best way for our communities. Very often, nurses feel inferior. Nurses expect to be inferior to other professions. We should not place ourselves in the position as a leader. Anyone in a community can be a leader. Leadership is not a program or training. It is a mind-set.

Three years ago when I received a leadership scholarship from the Florence Nightingale Foundation and Burdett Trust for Nurses, I enrolled into a couple of programs at the Royal Academy of Dramatic Arts in London. Through dramatic arts, I was enabled to develop myself with a focus in women-specific leadership—how to read yourself, how to get to know yourself, and what your personality preferences are. I realized that I was really quite shy when faced with opportunities to communicate with very senior professionals in government, especially women, so working on being a good communicator was vital. I worked with them to reach my equilibrium. I learned so much of who I am. My advice: Seek unusual experiences like this.

Other pieces of advice for nurses:

- Find a mentor or multiple mentors from a variety of sectors. Seek support and challenge outside nursing.
- Being positive attracts people. Sell your vision as you develop as a leader.
- Be business savvy. None of us can assume that money will keep coming and we will keep working. Nurses are creative but need to market themselves as that.
- We create armors around ourselves, but the future is about collaboration and leadership. In the words of Jeremy Scrivens, a social entrepreneur, collaboration is the new innovation! In my organization, we are thinking along the lines of the American Nurses Credentialing Center (ANCC) Magnet® model as a number of NHS Trusts are developing this or at least the principles. I am committed to developing person-centered programs and community assets models. We are advocates in our communities, and we know how to do this.

How did these opportunities come to you? What things did you consider before accepting these opportunities?

I have recently become confident enough to take myself out of my comfort zone. It's easy to be at a place where you know what you're doing and are the nurse consultant or deputy to the chief nurse, but being at the top of your game can be a little stifling if you don't push boundaries and seek external opportunities. Go into the unknown. Ask, "Will you help me?" One example concerns a CEO for a nursing charity and a nonnursing charity CEO, who is a nurse. They both wholeheartedly supported me to make the transition from government to the third sector. They both said, "You are ready to lead now." They saw something in me that excited them. They both now mentor me, and we have a great time together!

The charity sector in the United Kingdom is known as the third sector. Nurses are great at doing things the "third way," so we should be exploring this sector and looking to see where the gaps are. There is no reason why a nurse can't set up a charity or social enterprise.

How do I, 30 years into my career, support nurses in big organizations? My ethical and moral compass regarding leadership is to mentor across the next generation of nurses to support them to take risks. Actually, I have found that our millennial nurses and undergraduates are much more linked in to societal issues and planetary health. It's refreshing to talk with younger nurses about their ambitions. They are ambitious for our profession.

Through the many transitions you went through as you advanced in your career, what were your challenges? Did you have a certain degree of anxiety in stepping forward?

The biggest challenge and transition I can think of was as deputy chief nurse for Public Health England (PHE) as I moved to a national strategic leadership position literally overnight. I had a 3-year-old son and moved from a part-time to a full-time role, traveled a lot, and spent my days involved in very sensitive communication with key people nationally and internationally.

Very quickly, the Ebola outbreak happened in 2014, and I was responsible for leading critical aspects of the program for about 18 months. I was brought into the national team as a nurse adviser and also co-led the governance team. PHE provided staff to Sierra Leone and also provided teams to manage every airport and port of entry into England. I was propelled into a very serious situation very quickly.

Around 6 months into my job, I fell; I tanked. I lacked confidence. I wasn't sure of what I was doing. I was scared I was going to be found out as an impostor. My national director of human resources (HR) saw me and noted that I was not my usual self. My HR director asked me if I was okay. I said, "No, I'm not." Right there and then, she connected me with an executive coach. I worked with a coach for about 18 months, created a great bond, and had a fantastic relationship. My coach and I probably met about 10 times in 18 months and worked on my deep consciousness and deep-seated belief that I was an impostor, that I did not deserve it, and that it was pure luck and I had no skill or talent. We are still in touch and meet occasionally to reflect and check in. Now, it's my turn. I coach and mentor many nurses and undergraduates. I am also reverse mentored too by an early career nurse. This is very challenging but very beneficial for both of us, I hope!

Describe an example in your professional career where you felt you were at the right place, at the right time, and was totally prepared to embrace a new opportunity.

It's all about people and communication. When I was about 33, I had been in nursing about 15 years. I was within a role where I was quite autonomous but not enough. I worked with a population of refugees, asylum-seeking families, and unaccompanied children. I had a work partner, Karen, and we did a lot. I knew there was more to do. I wanted to do my MPH. At that time, my employer was a community NHS organization. I told my manager we need a nurse consultant here to lead and progress this nurse-led service. She said, "Not on my watch. We don't need nurse consultants here." I also asked if I could do my MPH. She asked why. I had to leave and went back to London to school to study part time for my MPH and went back to my previous employer, who was amazing and funded my studies and allocated me to a part-time case load in order to focus. I knew that by getting my MPH, it would get me to where I needed to be. In my MPH, I met people in public health. They took me to their work (like Centers for Disease Control and Prevention), and I was absolutely amazed with the level of autonomy and advanced level practice by nurse consultants in a historically medical and scientific environment. They saw I had a passion; a job opened and I applied. After a year, I had worked my way to be a nurse consultant in health protection, managed large outbreaks of measles, looked at policy changes, and made huge decisions that affected populations. People saw something in me and supported me to achieve my goals. Leadership in my team focused around the person or people we served and what outcome we required. Then skills and talents were sourced from the team. It didn't matter whether you were a nurse, doctor, or scientist. If you had the skills, you led. Simple as that.

What are you most proud of, professionally?

I proved everyone wrong. I was a square peg in a round hole. I left/ran from school at 16 with nothing and then went to college, enrolled on a prenursing course, and retook all my exams. I met teachers in college who treated me as a human and a grown-up and took exams in really exciting subjects such as sociology, human development, and psychology. When I went to college, people thought I would never be able to make it. I'm not for the academic stuff. I was told to go to a smaller district hospital to undertake my nursing training. I disagreed, pulled myself up, focused, and passed my exams. Life is based on early failures. Everything worth doing is worth working for. As William Rathbrone said, "What ought to be done, should be done."

Key Points

- Do not stagnate. Be prepared to embrace new experiences and opportunities.
- Examine where you are spending your energy and check that these are aligned to your individual development plan and organizational goals.
- Successful transition to a new manager position requires support through mentorship, preceptorship, and a formal orientation process.

References

American Organization for Nursing Leadership. (2015). *AONL nurse manager competencies*. Chicago, IL: AONL. Retrieved from https://www.aonl.org/system/files/media/file/2019/04/nurse-manager-competencies.pdf

Barnes, H. (2015). Exploring the factors that influence the nurse practitioner role transition. *Journal of Nurse Practice, 11*(2), 178–183. doi:10.1016/j.nurpra.2014.11.004

Bureau of Labor Statistics. (2016). *Job openings and labor turnover.* Washington, DC: US Department of Labor.

Center for Creative Leadership. (2019). Retrieved from ccl.org

Cross, R. (2019). To be happier at work, invest more in your relationships. *Harvard Business Review*. Retrieved from https://hbr.org/2019/07/to-be-happier-at-work-invest-more-in-your-relationships

Doria, H. (2015). Successful transition from staff nurse to manager. *Nurse Leader, 13*(1), 78–81. doi:10.1016/j.mnl.2014.07.013

Evans, L. (2019). *How to adjust after relocating for a job*. Retrieved from https://www.fastcompany.com/90294972/how-to-adjust-after-relocating-for-a-job

Forbes Coaches Council. (2016). 12 Pitfalls when moving from mid-to upper-level management. *Forbes*. Retrieved from https://www.forbes.com/sites/forbescoachescouncil/2016/11/03/when-mid-management-becomes-upper-level-management-how-to-support-this-transition/#8efc3f54a315

Hackensack University Medical Center. (2019). *Designed to recognize and motivate ongoing development of expertise and professionalism of our nurses*. Retrieved from https://www.hackensackumc.org/nursing/professional-development/clinical-ladders/

Hoffman, R. L., Klein, S. J., & Rosenzweig, M. Q. (2017). Creating quality online materials for specialty nurse practitioner content: Filling a need for the graduate nurse practitioner. *Journal of Cancer Education, 32*(3), 522–527. doi:10.1007/s13187-015-0980-3

Kalwacki, E., Fellman, J., & Torosian, J. (2015). A nursing recognition program gets a makeover. *American Nurse Today, 10*(1). Retrieved from https://dev01.americannursetoday.com/nursing-recognition-program-gets-makeover/

Loyola University Health System. (2013). *Clinical ladder guidelines*. Retrieved from http://www.luhs.org/feature/nursing/Clinical_Ladder/CLGUIDLN%209.09_1.pdf

Marten, J., Motz, J., & Stump, L. (2018). A certified registered nurse anesthetist's transition to manager. *American Association of Nurse Anesthetists, 86*(6), 448–454.

Minsky, L., & Peter, J. T. (2019). Are your at risk of a mid-career rut? *Harvard Business Review*. Retrieved from https://hbr.org/2019/09/are-you-at-risk-of-a-mid-career-rut?ab=hero-subleft-1

Moss, C., & Jackson, J. (2019). Mentoring new graduate nurse practitioners. *Neonatal Network, 38*(3), 151–159. doi:10.1891/0730-0832.38.3.151

Paige, L. (2015). *10 ways for nurses to get promoted*. Retrieved from https://minoritynurse.com/10-ways-for-nurses-to-get-promoted/

Pilat, M., & Merriam, D. H. (2019). Exploring the lived experiences of staff nurses transitioning to the nurse manager role. *The Journal of Nursing Administration, 49*(10), 509–513. doi:10.1097/NNA.0000000000000795.

Raso, R. (2013). Brace yourself: Leaving your comfort zone. *Nursing Management, 44*(8), 6. Retrieved from https://journals.lww.com/nursingmanagement/fulltext/2013/08000/Brace_yourself__Leaving_your_comfort_zone.1.aspx

Sheikhib, M., Fallahi-Khoshnab, M., Mohammadi, F., & Oskouie, F. (2016). Skills required for nursing career advancement: A qualitative study. *Nursing and Midwifery Studies, 5*(2), e30777. doi:10.17795/nmsjournal30777

Wiggins, A. (2017). Setting yourself up for success in a new organization. *Nursing Management, 48*(11), 52–54. Retrieved from https://journals.lww.com/nursingmanagement/FullText/2017/11000/Setting_yourself_up_for_success_in_a_new.12.aspx

Zastocki, D. (2010). *Retaining nurse managers.* Retrieved from https://www.americannursetoday.com/retaining-nurse-managers/

4

Being Involved: What's in It for Me?

Rhoda R. Redulla

"From there, I became the Chair of the Nursing Quality and Patient Safety Council, championing the hospital's efforts to reduce CAUTI and CLABSI rates."

—Patrick Lallier, MPA, BSN, RN, CCRN

This chapter covers the almost endless possibilities to be involved within an organization, within a professional nursing organization, and within the community.

Whenever I meet with new nurses, I always say that the best advice I can give them is to join a committee or participate in a project and get involved—a new program that is being rolled out by the hospital, a product that is being replaced, or a new process that is being implemented. The possibilities are endless for nurses to participate in performance or quality improvement. Nurse leaders are always looking for team members to facilitate or assist in projects at the unit, department, or organizational levels. And for me, being involved is the perfect opportunity to give back to the profession and serve patients and families while developing my leadership skills and confidence.

The American Nurses Credentialing Center (ANCC) Magnet® model supports and promotes professional development. Organizations that are working toward Magnet designation or those that have achieved the designation are required to support the professional development of nurses. The Magnet model has set the framework to allow nurses to advance professionally. Embedded in the model is the "Structural

Empowerment" domain (ANCC, 2019). Magnet-recognized organizations use multiple strategies to create structures and processes that support a lifelong learning culture that includes professional collaboration and promotion of role development, academic achievement, and career advancement (ANCC, 2019).

Furthermore, nurses who are retained in a Magnet-recognized hospital are involved directly in making choices in patient care, and they are active in contributing to health-care changes based on evidence-based practice (EBP; Flaugher, Beyea, & Slattery, 2015).

PROFESSIONAL (SHARED) GOVERNANCE

Porter-O'Grady and Finnigan (1984) defined shared governance as a professional practice model founded on the cornerstone principles of partnership, equity, accountability, and ownership that form a culturally sensitive and empowering framework, enabling sustainable and accountability-based decisions to support an interdisciplinary design for excellent patient care. Individual organizations have developed their own definition of shared governance, aligned with these principles. Vanderbilt University Medical Center (VUMC), one of the first hospitals in the nation to implement shared governance, defines shared governance as a dynamic staff–leader partnership that promotes collaboration, shared decision-making, and accountability for improving quality of care, safety, and enhancing work–life balance. In 2016, Clavelle, Porter O'Grady, Weston, and Verran (2016) recommended the shift from "shared governance" to "professional governance."

BEING INVOLVED: WITHIN THE ORGANIZATION

Nursing was one of the first professions in healthcare to implement shared governance and VUMC (n.d.) was one of the first hospitals that adopted the shared governance model. The following venues reflect shared governance: unit councils, work groups, task forces, process improvement teams, operations councils, practice committees, and so forth.

Unit Council

The unit council is the basic unit of professional or shared governance in a healthcare organization. It is a decision-making body led by a unit council chair, with several unit council members. The group typically meets monthly. Most organizations have a professional governance model and establish guidelines to guide unit councils. Unit councils identify the strategic goals of the unit, aligned with the strategic priorities of the organization. A hospital sets the strategic priority of decreasing healthcare-associated infections (HAIs). The current state of HAIs shows opportunities to improve central line associated bloodstream infection (CLABSI) and *Clostridium difficile* infection. The unit council then examines its own data and identifies goals for the unit. For example, in the surgical intensive care unit (SICU), the CLABSI rates were above target for the past 2 consecutive months. The unit council then identifies this as a priority area to work on and creates an action plan to lower the CLABSI rates. The action plan may include reviewing the current protocol for central line dressing and tubing changes, developing a checklist to ensure nurses are maintaining a closed system, and providing education to the team.

How can you get involved? Based on the set strategic goals of the unit, individual members work together to achieve the desired outcomes. If you are a unit council member, this is your opportunity to lead, co-lead, or support a unit initiative. From the planned CLABSI quality improvement initiative, you can volunteer to lead or help champion it. In the process, you develop your skills in EBP, communication, and innovation. Your involvement in the CLABSI work group could be the beginning of a career in nursing quality and performance improvement. Nursing quality specialists apply data management and analytic skills to identify opportunities to improve healthcare delivery, including patient safety and performance improvement. Nursing quality specialists gather data and identify patterns and trends in various clinical indicators such as readmissions, infections, and patient falls. These quality experts can advance in leadership roles such as director of nursing quality and/or patient safety. Your experience in participating in unit-based initiatives can create connections for you to explore other career opportunities within nursing and to advance professionally.

Department-Wide and Organization-Wide Committees

Inherent to the professional governance model are the department-wide and organization-wide committees. Again, this opens up more opportunities for nurses to participate in various quality or performance improvement projects. The structure of both department-wide and organization-wide committees is determined by each organization.

The following are examples of these committees in nursing:

- Nursing practice
- Nursing quality and safety

- Nursing research, EBP, and innovation
- Nursing professional development
- Nursing recognition, recruitment, and retention (R3)
- Nursing informatics

These committees typically report to a campus-wide nursing committee, represented by the chair. Figure 4.1 presents an example of a professional governance structure. At the core of the model is the unit-based councils. Designated members represent the unit council in the campus-wide councils, such as the nurse practice council and nurse quality council. Depending on the structure set by the organization, chairs from all campus-wide committees can meet at the nursing coordinating council, or all unit council chairs can also be part of the bigger council.

The SICU's work on CLABSI prevention can be replicated and adopted by other inpatient units across the department. It could also be the offshoot of a major quality improvement initiative at the organizational level.

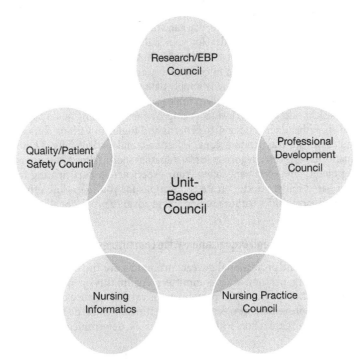

Figure 4.1 Nursing coordinating council.

EBP, evidence-based practice.

Organization-Wide Committee

An organization-wide committee is composed of members from interprofessional teams (multiple disciplines) such as pharmacy, laboratory, physical therapy and rehabilitation, food and nutrition, security, and information technology. Various committees are established to meet the operational and strategic goals of the organization.

Here are examples of organization-wide committees:

- Medication safety committee
- Blood utilization committee
- Patient flow committee
- Zero harm committee
- Budget/finance committee
- Community outreach committee
- Infection prevention committee

These committees present additional opportunities for nurses to make an impact in creating a positive work environment and patient outcomes. Let's talk about the work of the medication safety committee as an example. Adverse drug events (ADE) are one of the leading causes of significant harm and death among hospitalized patients and relate to any unintentional harm to a patient caused by drug use, misuse, or nonuse (Phillips et al., 2014). An ADE is defined as an injury or harm resulting from medical intervention related to a drug. The primary aim of the committee is to ensure safe administration of medications and prevent harm. The functions of the committee include formulating and reviewing policies related to medication administration, reviewing adverse events related to medication administration, developing advisories on changes in medication delivery devices, and proposing alternatives during drug shortages. Nursing representatives provide perspective on the nurses' workflow, feedback on revisions in policies and procedures, and so on. An example is, during a certain period, an increase in the incidence of needle sticks related to SC insulin administration was noted. The input of nurses on this observation is important as the medication safety committee drafts solutions to address issues related to the observation. Clinical nurses may share concerns on the syringe product currently used and workflow issues that predispose nurses to injuries. Nurses can champion developing a survey to obtain nursing input on needle stick prevention. Needle stick injuries can present a multitude of issues, including possible lost work time and emotional impact to the affected nurse. This is another illustration on how being involved in a committee creates a notable impact in the organization. Still within the medication safety committee, nurses provide insight during drug shortages. This can mean substituting a medication that comes in a larger dose, such as an

IV antibiotic, for example, with multiple smaller doses. Nurses can comment whether the proposed change is feasible from a workflow perspective and present alternative solutions if not.

Another great example is the shift to a new electronic medical record (EMR). Who are the experts in determining the steps in documentation? How can the EMR be designed to provide cost-effective care? Clinical nurses provide critical information in developing the EMR. My current organization is transitioning to a new EMR. In addition to the formal meetings related to the build process, the manager for nursing informatics presented an update to a group of clinical nurses. You will be surprised at the numerous questions that nurses have, with a trail of "What ifs…" and "What is the plan for.…" Nurses are familiar with the workflow and seem to always have a third eye on what could not work in the clinical arena. It was great seeing nurses passionately advocating for how the system should be designed and kept, and asking how and why throughout the presentation.

Work Group/Task Force

The changes happening in healthcare or even just in an organization sometimes affect the progress of some initiatives. When this happens, or when, for any reason, the organization is lagging behind on its goals, a special work group or task force may be convened.

Hourly Rounding Example

At one hospital, the patient experience score on nurse communication was poor. At the beginning of the year, an educational series was completed based on communication standards that were established. Included in the series were topics on active listening, verbal and nonverbal communication, and so on. After all nurses completed the course, a slight increase was noted in the patient experience score on nurse communication. However, in the third quarter, a decline in the score began and continued to drop steadily month by month. The nurse leaders from the medical-surgical units noted that the affected units were mostly their areas. Preliminary comments obtained from various units showed that there was an inconsistency in the hourly rounding practice. Some nurses were following the guidelines, while some were skipping some steps. Other nurses were not doing it at all. Hourly rounding is an evidence-based intervention geared toward improving nurse–patient communication, fall prevention, and prevention of hospital-acquired pressure injuries and other hospital-acquired conditions. The identified need of improving the nurse communication Hospital Consumer Assessment of Healthcare Providers and Systems (HCAHPS) score led to the development of a task force. How does a task force differ from a committee?

Differences Between a Committee and Task Force

A committee is the most formal of the work groups. It is composed of groups of persons appointed or selected to perform a function on behalf of a larger group. A task force is a small group of individuals brought together to address a specific objective (Grigsby, 2008).

SUCCESS STORY

Patrick Lallier, MPA, BSN, RN, CCRN

Administrative Nursing Supervisor,
University of North Carolina (UNC) Health Care, Chapel Hill, North Carolina

Patrick is currently a patient care director of the ambulatory surgery, postanesthesia care unit (PACU), and surgical short-stay units at NewYork-Presbyterian/Weill Cornell Medical Center (NYP/WC). In this role, Patrick oversees a team of approximately 65 employees, including nurse practitioners, clinical nurses, nursing assistants, perioperative patient assistants, and business associates. Leading the team consists of strategizing, developing action plans to target specific challenges or goals, and supporting staff in their own development, engagement, and, at times, corrective action.

What was your success story about being involved in committee work?

I first became involved in committee work as a clinical support technician, prior to starting my nursing career at NYP/WC. As a clinical support tech, I was passionate about career advancement and helped found the assistive personnel career advancement team at UNC Medical Center, a campus-wide initiative to engage support staff in furthering their education or gaining new skills that would support the institution. When I arrived at NYP/WC, I quickly joined the unit council on the surgical stepdown unit, serving first as secretary and then as the representative on the nursing quality and patient safety (NQPS) council—a hospital-wide committee with the goal of helping to reduce hospital-acquired infections and patient falls. From there I became the chair of the NQPS council, championing the hospital's efforts to reduce catheter-associated urinary tract infection (CAUTI) and central line associated bloodstream infection (CLASBI) rates. This work led up to the creation of the hospital's first-ever Healthcare-Associated Infection (HAI) Champions program. The HAI Champions program initially started as a CLABSI reduction team. Related to this work, I joined the Magnet® document writing team, specifically the exemplary practice arm of the team, and authored and coauthored three narratives for the NYP/WC Magnet document.

What is your advice for fellow nurses?

I would advise nurses who are just starting their careers to sink their teeth into becoming the best clinical nurse they can be—find ways to expand their professional knowledge and skills, such as continuing education or certification; reflect on your personal strengths and lean toward those strengths as you plan your career path; and look at ways to address your opportunities for improvement. Finally, I would recommend getting the highest degree you are able to afford and that also aligns with your career goals. This year I finished my master's in public administration with a focus on nursing leadership, and the skills I gained from that experience have already proved extremely valuable in this work.

What are you most proud of?

In reflecting on my year and one-half of nursing leadership experience, I would say I am most proud of the relationship I developed with my staff, built on the foundation of empathy and respect. I am also proud of the challenges I have overcome, including a difficult transition when one of my units was divided to create a brand-new hospital unit—the team building and conflict resolution skills it took to achieve that transition without major turnover were significant, and it was definitely a validating experience.

BENEFITS OF BEING INVOLVED

By participating in projects or increasing your involvement in committee work, unit or department activities, your leadership skills are developed and you advance your knowledge and practice. The most important outcome is the opportunity to influence the care you give to your patients and advance the nursing profession while creating connections with peers and mentors.

What Could Be Stopping Nurses From Getting Involved?

Nurses can name several reasons why they do not join in committee work. Some of these can seem so simple yet so real in the healthcare setting.

Lack of Time

Regardless of the setting, on most days pulling away from your normal responsibilities to attend a committee meeting is almost impossible. During peak times during the shift, nurses can hardly find time to take a bathroom break, let alone attend an hour-long meeting. Sometimes, the unit has planned the staffing to include a buffer in staffing coverage when a nurse leaves for a meeting. However, emergencies can occur at the last minute and preclude the nurse from attending the meeting. In one article, Domrose cited the experience of one nurse who had no plans to join a committee and wondered how she would fit a monthly meeting into her schedule. "Truthfully, I joined because no one else volunteered," she said. After her involvement in the committee and developing her skills as a leader, the nurse became an assistant manager.

The Solution

Making professional (shared) governance involvement thrive requires a mutual commitment between the organization and individual nurses (Domrose, 2011). Do you have "protected meeting time" at your work? As nurses commit to devoting their time in committee work, organizations extend support by providing what is known as protected meeting time. Some organizations create dedicated cost centers so time spent on meetings are accounted for and are not coded as direct nursing care hours. Otherwise, attendance to meetings can impact the unit's productivity level. The time required to be physically present at the meetings is just one. Once nurses are involved in a project, they also need more time to do committee-related work, such as preparing the meeting agenda, collecting data, and developing educational materials.

Not Sure of What to Contribute

Nurses can be stuck thinking that they do not have anything new to contribute or that they need to know the answers when they join a committee. Or worse, nurses are afraid that they will say the wrong words and cause confusion. When it was Zinnia's, a former colleague, first time to participate in a committee, she confessed that she did not say anything for the first three meetings, except when she introduced herself at the beginning of each meeting. Zinnia joined the hand hygiene committee. First, she was nervous and was not really too keen about speaking in front of a group. Zinnia observed the other members of the committee and noted that most of them were really just sharing on what was the current state of the hand hygiene program in their respective units. Another member narrated his most recent conversation with a patient on his perspective of the hand hygiene process at the hospital. Other times, the committee chair would ask for group recommendations, and Zinnia also noticed that not everyone needed to have an answer. By the fourth month, she went to the meeting prepared. The committee members were asked to report on their unit's hand hygiene compliance data. This effectively broke the tense mind-set she was in during the meetings. A few months after, guess what? Zinnia found herself leading an audit task force within the committee!

The Solution

Speak with a current committee member, or ask the chair to pair you up with an experienced member. Be familiar with the current priorities of the committee and actively seek out information on how you can best contribute. Ask advice from your manager. Devote part of your midyear or annual performance review to discuss your goals and specific needs about being an active member of a committee or initiative.

Lack of Manager Support

In my experience working with nurses, not having the full support and guidance of a manager has come up as a legitimate barrier in being involved. This can turn out to be a major deterrent for nurses who are just starting to build their motivation and skills to participate in quality improvement or in the broad agenda of the unit or department. Without a supportive environment, it is easy for nurses to feel either reluctant or intimidated to approach their managers. I have also seen highly engaged nurses who decided to stop being involved because of lack of support from their managers. How do nurses sense that their managers are not supportive of their involvement in committees or initiatives? Nurses in these situations have shared some examples, such as their requests to meet with the manager may not be given priority or there is no response to emails requesting to support a project.

The Solution

Managers set the tone for the importance of being involved in committees and initiatives. After all, with a well-engaged frontline staff, managers' jobs become a lot easier. However, when managers are at different phases of development in an organization, it is helpful to establish communication guidelines. The guidelines outline the frequency of communication, and it needs to be specific, for example, in-person, monthly meeting. Another best practice is to have a collective retreat for frontline nurses (e.g., unit council chairs) and managers and have them both sign a commitment form. The commitment form outlines the role expectations from both the manager and the staff in terms of committee involvement.

What's in It for Me?

I have a simple answer to this question: because you would like to be the best nurse and professional you can be for your patients and their families and for colleagues. By being involved, you learn new ideas, meet new people, and grasp new strategies and better ways to do things. What's in it for you? It's actually your gift to you!

BEING INVOLVED: IN A PROFESSIONAL NURSING ORGANIZATION

Last year, I gave a talk on advancing in your professional journey. I used a metaphor to illustrate the importance of joining a professional organization. I invited the audience to visualize a basket of fruits that a friend hands to you to share with others or eat some of them yourself. Instead of sharing or eating the fruits, you put them on the kitchen counter. I asked what happens if you just leave them on the kitchen counter or forget about them. The fruits become moldy and rotten, right? The same happens with our nursing profession. When you don't nurture it through your contributions and involvement or take the time to share your skills, knowledge, and expertise with your nursing colleagues, then our profession could fail or die. Abigail Schneider (2015) explained thus: "How do nursing organizations fit in with my professional development? The answer is simple: Nursing organizations may very well be the backbone of professional development." And I add, one's effort to engage in professional development is one of the backbones of the nursing profession.

Professional Nursing Organizations

Each organization offers a myriad of opportunities to become involved. These are anchored in the organization's mission and agenda. As of 2012, there are over 100 national nursing organizations (Matthews, 2012).

American Nurses Association

The American Nurses Association (ANA) is the premier organization representing the interests of the 4 million RNs in the United States. The ANA was founded in 1896 and has members in all 50 states and U.S. territories. The organization is considered the strongest voice of the profession (ANA, 2018).

According to the ANA (2010), "professional development is a vital phase of lifelong learning in which nurses engage to develop and maintain competence, enhance professional nursing practice, and support achievement of career goals."

The ANA achieves its mission to advance the nursing profession by fostering high standards of nursing practice. The organization provides direction for nurses by providing a framework for professional nursing practice. The ANA ensures that these standards of practice are current and relevant to nurses and address the needs of every practice setting.

ANA Nursing Standards

The scope and standards of practice resources describe the art and science of nursing and the details associated with specialty nursing practice.

ANA Position Statements

When a hot topic arises in the industry, the ANA will create an explanation, justification, or recommendation for a course of action—otherwise known as a position statement.

ANA Principles for Nursing Practice

From pay to staffing, delegation to documentation, and even for cutting-edge topics such as social media, the ANA has principles aimed at giving nurses practical information for their professional practice.

Here are some principles created by the ANA:

- Principles for Advanced Practice Registered Nurse (APRN) Full Practice Authority
- Principles of Collaborative Relationships
- Principles for Social Networking and the Nurse
- Principles for Pay for Quality
- Principles for Nurse Staffing
- Core Principles on Connected Health

You can access more information on the ANA Principles for nursing practice here: https://www.nursingworld.org/practice-policy/nursing-excellence/official-position-statements/ana-principles/.

How to Be Involved

To help carry out its mission through each of the strategies mentioned, the ANA invites nurse volunteers to participate in various committees, work panels, and groups. The ANA sends out an annual call for willingness to serve. On the ANA website, there is a section on "Get involved." Here, nurses can obtain information on how to advocate, connect, share their expertise, or donate to existing projects of the organization.

- Advocate via political action committees and RN action committees: Connect with the ANA community, ANA Capitol Beat, and Magnet Learning communities and Pathway to Excellence communities, specific to the ANCC Magnet Recognition Program and Pathway to Excellence.
- Share your expertise as an ANA professional issues panel or subject matter expert. There are also many opportunities

throughout the year, such as serving as an abstract reviewer for the ANA conferences. The national conferences include the ANCC Magnet® conference, ANCC Pathway to Excellence, and the ANA Quality and Innovation Quality conference. Another opportunity is to serve as moderator or facilitator during the conference.

American Academy of Critical-Care Nurses

The American Academy of Critical-Care Nurses (AACN) has over 100,000 members comprising a community of acute and critical care nurses. On its website (https://www.aacn.org/nursing-excellence/volunteers/ambassadors/become-an-ambassador), the AACN has outlined the benefits of becoming an AACN member: unlimited free continuing education opportunities; access to award-winning journals, clinical toolkits, and evidence-based resources; innovative and evidence-based programs; and discounts for conferences and educational events.

Every year, over 1,000 nurses volunteer to the AACN. AACN members generously contribute their time to help influence, shape, and define the practice of critical care nursing and the healthcare profession. When you volunteer, you add to your professional growth by networking with a wide range of skilled peers and developing your leadership skills (aacn.org).

Advisory Teams

Advisory teams provide feedback on specific issues and related strategies regarding AACN initiatives. These groups are issue driven and are based on specific professional expertise depending on group content. These groups take part in an online discussion database or communicate via email where participants explore significant issues from the convenience of their home or workplace.

While these groups may be expected to participate in conference calls or may be called upon to respond to written manuals and materials, the bulk of work will take place via the Internet through the volunteer database or via email. Past advisory teams included staff nurses, nurse managers, and progressive care nurses.

Ambassadors

When you become an ambassador, you enter into a dynamic partnership with the national component of our AACN community that strengthens over time based on learning on both sides. You agree to fulfill your role obligations to the best of your ability and in keeping with the mission and values of the association.

In exchange, the national staff agrees to uphold its obligations to support the ambassadors in optimally fulfilling their role obligations and to enhance its support over time.

AACN Ambassador Accountabilities

- Actively promote the AACN in your unit and/or facility, including communicating the value of the AACN to staff nurses and nursing leadership.
- Stay up to date on AACN initiatives and forward relevant information to your colleagues using key resources such as *AACN Bold Voices*, *Critical Care Nurse*, *American Journal of Critical Care*, CriticalCare Newsline, and the AACN website.
- Respond to communication from the AACN by the stated deadline or within 1 week if no deadline is specified.
- Participate in online forums provided by the national staff to ensure networking of ambassadors.
- Partner with local chapters to advance AACN initiatives within your community.
- Join review panels and certification, publishing, and task force groups.

Think Tanks

Think tanks are leadership groups that are directly linked to the National Office work spheres, addressing issues that impact functional departments such as practice, research, certification, professional development, membership, chapters, and volunteer services.

These groups identify and evaluate global trends and issues, in turn strategizing and making new suggestions for the future of the Association and the healthcare profession. Think tanks require travel one or two times a year and may participate in one or two conference calls that can be taken from home or work.

Oncology Nursing Society

The Oncology Nursing Society is the premier organization for oncology nursing with over 39,000 members. On its website, the "Make a Difference" heading covers all the relevant information on how to get involved:

- Join your local chapter
- Join our communities
- Join the mentor program
- Volunteer
- Become an abstract reviewer
- Join the CJON Editorial Board
- Join the CJON Review Board
- Join the Congress planning team
- Join the International Review Panel

The ANA is one of more than 100 national nursing organizations (Matthews, 2012). Nursing organizations such as the ANA and the National League for Nursing (NLN) have a broad focus, encompassing the entire nursing profession, whereas organizations such as the AACN, the Society of Pediatric Nurses, the National Association of Orthopedic Nurses, and others are focused on disease processes (diabetes, renal, cardiac), healthcare settings (hospital, clinic, surgical), age (pediatrics, geriatrics), or advanced practice (clinical nurse specialists, nurse executives, nurse educators; Matthews, 2012).

Academy of Medical-Surgical Nursing

The Academy of Medical-Surgical Nurses (AMSN) is the only specialty nursing organization dedicated to the practice of medical-surgical nursing. The AMSN's mission is to promote excellence in medical-surgical nursing (www.amsn.org). It has almost 12,000 members, and its certification affiliate, the Medical-Surgical Nursing Certification Board, has over 28,500 nurses certified and using the CMSRN credential and the care coordination and transition management CCCTM credential.

The AMSN presents many opportunities for nurses to be involved. It has a robust volunteer units program devoted to:

- Improving patient care
- Developing personally and professionally
- Advocating for the specialty of medical-surgical nursing
- Connecting with other nurses who share their compassion and commitment

The AMSN volunteer units include Ambassadors, the AMSN PRISM Awards Committee, Clinical Practice, Legislative, MedSurg Newsletter, Nominating, NAQC, Program Planning, Research Coordinator and Team, Scholarship and Awards.

Some of these volunteer units are highlighted in the following:

- Clinical Practice addresses issues that pertain to clinical practice in medical-surgical nursing, by expanding the awareness and utilization of EBP, and performance/quality improvement among medical-surgical nurses. These issues range from pain management to delegation.
- Program Planning coordinates the AMSN Annual Convention, the premier medical-surgical nursing conference. Program Planning members determine the educational offerings.
- The Scholarship and Awards Committee promotes, coordinates, and administers $40,000 in scholarships, grants, and awards annually, aligned with the AMSN's mission to promote excellence in medical-surgical nursing.

American Academy of Ambulatory Care Nursing

The American Academy of Ambulatory Care Nursing (AAACN) is the professional organization and community for RNs in all ambulatory care settings. It is 3,000 RN-members strong, all of whom practice in ambulatory care settings such as hospital-based outpatient clinics/centers, independent/group medical practices, telehealth call centers, university hospitals, community hospitals, military and Veterans Affairs (VA) settings, managed care/health maintenance organizations (HMOs)/preferred provider organizations (PPOs), colleges/educational institutions, patient homes, and free-standing facilities.

Here are more examples of professional nursing organizations. You can also find a more comprehensive list on this website: https://nurse.org/orgs.shtml.

- American Academy of Nurse Practitioners
- National Association of Critical-Care Nurses
- Oncology Nursing Society
- National Association of Orthopedic Nurses
- American Nephrology Nurses Association
- Society of Gastroenterology Nurses and Associates
- Society of Pediatric Nurses
- Wound Ostomy and Continence Nurses Society

What's in It for Me?

You may be asking yourself: What's in it for me? How do nursing organizations fit in with my professional development? Your membership in a nursing organization unites you with your peers. When nurses unite, we have a much stronger voice in the political arena on local, state, and national levels. Remember when the hosts of a daytime talk show created controversy after they made light of nursing as a valued profession.? Nurses united, took a stand, and spoke in one voice, and as a result, the show issued an official apology. The ANA (2015) issued a statement in which the response of the nursing community was validated, and the apology was accepted.

Membership in a professional nursing organization provides nurses with continuing education, certification opportunities, role-related competencies, and educational conferences. Changes in healthcare occur almost daily. Aligning with a nursing organization that supports your specialty or population of practice positions nurses to be on the forefront of practice changes. Nursing organizations promote and encourage the use of EBP to its members. Nurses who are certified in their specialty will find that their nursing professional organization will offer continuing education that is pertinent to their practice. Many nursing organizations hold annual nursing conferences that bring nurses together from across the country and often from around the world, to share education and best practices. They also offer the opportunity to network with nursing colleagues from around the globe.

- Committee work
- Elected officer (president, board member)
- Committee chair or member
- Types of committees
- Task force

SUCCESS STORY

Courtney Ruck, MSN, RN, SCRN

Nursing Unit Director, T2, Reading Hospital at Tower Health, Reading, Pennsylvania

Currently I am the patient care director for the neuroscience step-down unit and the Interventional Neuroradiology Unit at NewYork-Presbyterian/Weill Cornell (NYP/WC) Medical Center. In this role, I manage the nursing and ancillary personnel of each unit as well as the daily patient operations to ensure we are delivering safe, efficient patient- and family-centered care.

What helped you achieve your current professional status?

The biggest driver that helped me accomplish and achieve my current professional status was through mentorship by my former patient care director. I always knew I wanted to pursue an advanced degree, but I was unsure of which track. Without the guidance and advice from my mentor, I would not be where I am today. Having a professional mentor allowed me (and still allows me) to ask questions, bounce around ideas, and gain better insights into what I want to accomplish and the best way to accomplish those goals throughout my professional nursing career.

Were you involved in committee work? If so, why did you get involved? Describe your experience, including some of your accomplishments.

During my professional career at NYP/WC, I became very involved in unit- and hospital-based committees. I began my committee journey by being the co-chair of my unit council, which led to chair of the council as well as chair of the hospital-wide recruitment, retention, and recognition (R3) council and the operations council. I wanted to join committees not only to improve the care of patients on the unit but also to help my professional development. Through my involvement in committees, I was able to help with unit-level changes as well as hospital-level changes. One achievement I worked on was creating an application for joining the unit council, which included an attestation of participation. This was rolled out on my unit due to a lack of attendance and participation by members as the year went on. It turned out to be so successful that it was rolled out hospital wide at NYP/WC Medical Center, with units tailoring the application to meet their needs.

What is your advice for nurses who are just starting in their nursing careers?

Become involved in anything and everything you're interested in! It is the best time when you're just starting out to try new things and see what path might be the best for you as you continue on your professional development journey. Meeting new people, generating new ideas to impact patient care, and continuing to advance the nursing profession are only a small number of amazing things you can do when you become involved in your organization.

BEING INVOLVED: IN THE COMMUNITY

Community outreach or community service may be viewed as just another extracurricular activity by some people. In healthcare, it can bring many life-changing moments to the patients and families served. Through service in the community, nurses have an opportunity to see the patient in the whole continuum of care, including the most vulnerable time after discharge from the hospital. In some cases, nurses may not realize the impact of small initiatives in the community. For example, acute care nurses' involvement in population-specific advocacy and community work, such as taxi driver and domestic worker health fairs in my current institution, can go a long way in preventing ED visits in these populations. Health fairs conducted by nurses can also improve adherence to the treatment regimen and prevent readmissions. Conducting coat drives and distributing gloves and thermals to vulnerable groups in the winter can prevent hospital admissions due to hypothermic emergencies. These initiatives look so simple and yet are quite eye-opening to our nurses when they realize many vulnerable groups in the community do not have access to basic healthcare.

How can nurses get involved?

Most organizations have either a community outreach committee or a community affairs office that sets the agenda for outreach activities.

The organization usually aligns their efforts based on a community service plan in the local areas served. Opportunities to be involved in various community outreach activities are released regularly.

In one organization, some outreach activities are conducted: free health screening and referral, health education such as cardiopulmonary resuscitation (CPR), serving in soup kitchens, distributing health-maintenance and health-promotion items. Department-specific outreach activities are also planned, which allow for more opportunities to partner with patients and families outside of the usual setting. An example is the outreach activity by the NewYork-Presbyterian/Weill Cornell Medical Center Oncology Division at a local Ronald McDonald House. The Ronald McDonald House is committed to providing shelter to family members during the hospitalization of a patient. Many oncology patients require long-term hospital stays. Oncology nurses establish meaningful partnerships with nonprofit organizations to improve the quality of life of patients and families and the overall patient experience. These are all opportunities for nurses to be involved in a highly rewarding activity. In the process, they develop new skills, meet new people, and expand their professional network.

Early in my career, I had been involved in many community outreach activities. I served as a volunteer instructor for the Red Cross teaching expectant mothers on preparing for delivery. I recall being very committed and passionate pursuing this outreach work. In the process, I developed my communication skills and embraced every new opportunity to be involved more. After a year of being an instructor, I was asked to participate in the training of trainers at the national level. I did not expect this opportunity to come to at all and learned a lot from it.

What Nurses Bring to Community Outreach

"We have a lot to learn from nurses," says Consuelo Wilkins (2018), executive director for the Meharry-Vanderbilt Alliance. Nurses are very important to community outreach and community involvement in healthcare. Wilkins does a lot of work with community-engaged health research, and if she sees a community engagement program that does not involve nurses, she comments, "They're not doing it right." Wilkins added that in most communities, nurses are much more embedded in the community than physicians and researchers or others in the healthcare system have ever been. She urged to put value in some of the frameworks and infrastructure that have been put in place by nurses. We really do need to tap into those resources, and they should be at the table leading a lot of this.

Nurse leaders are urged to pursue caring approaches that span the full healthcare continuum. This covers experiences before, during, and after hospitalization. Community outreach presents this opportunity while improving individual and population health outcomes. Nurses who are involved in community outreach seize a different kind of fulfillment. The implementation of the Patient Protection and Affordable Care Act (ACA) has further raised the expectation for organizations to demonstrate caring outcomes and ensure a structure where nurses practice to the full extent of their professional ability. In an article, Dyess, Opalinski, Saiswick, and Fox (2016) outlined questions for nurse leaders to consider when exploring opportunities for community outreach involvement:

- What are the current services and resources across the continuum of healthcare in the community?
- What services and resources are missing in our community?
- What service and resource opportunities can be realized?
- How is care provided for patients upon discharge posthospitalization, day 1, week 1, month 1, and beyond? Who are community caregivers (formal and informal)?
- Who are the constituents (primary caring/secondary caring)?
- With whom might innovative partnerships be formed?

These questions point to the significance of community outreach and the opportunities for nurses to make a difference in the community. The tremendous role of nurses in engaging the community is recognized.

The practice partner provides an established and extraordinary outreach program to the community as part of an organizational mission. Population health is addressed as part of this outreach. Health outcomes are measured, statistics are reported, and ongoing efforts are coordinated as part of a goal to improve the health of the area's residents. The practice partner regularly and actively reinvests within the geographic service area to improve access and navigation to the appropriate level of healthcare services. Efforts are made to provide community-based wellness and health education and to ensure the availability of charitable caring. Integrity, reverence, justice, commitment to the poor, and stewardship are the core values and the foundation for the community outreach that engages thousands of community members through community programs. Community outreach programs are located in elementary schools, faith communities, public libraries, parks, child daycare facilities, homeless venues, community agencies, and senior activity centers. The accomplishments and outcomes of the programs are partly due to the diverse partnerships established with local organizations, civic groups, key informant leaders, and other healthcare professionals. Initiatives are informed by knowledge of the need to address social determinants of well-being such as hunger, housing, literacy, and health disparities. Other health-related programming addresses chronic illness management, childhood and adult immunizations, and childhood obesity and fitness. HIV and hepatitis C virus infection counseling, testing, and linkage to care; school health, a comprehensive breast health program; and healthcare for individuals who are experiencing homelessness are part of the outreach endeavor. Key contributing factors lending to the success of this practice partner can be attributed to the hospital's support; a passionate, compassionate, and dedicated multidisciplinary staff team; and the earned trust of the community (Dyess et al., 2016, p. 142).

Nurses Share Why They Get Involved in Community Outreach

Burn Camp
Burn School Reentry, Pediatric Burn Support Group
Sylvia Dao, MS, MPA, RN, NE-BC

"We know our work doesn't start or stop at the hospital. It is important for us to be connected to our community to help prevent burns through education and support."

HIV Care, Testing and Prevention (Education, HIV/AIDS Walk)
Martha Mosco, BSN, RN, ACRN

"I love working for health and well-being in our larger communities. It always reminds me of the bigger picture of what we do and why. We get the opportunity to help people connect to healthcare and gain confidence to care for themselves."

Key Points

- Participating in a committee or being involved in an initiative is highly rewarding. It contributes to your professional development.
- Expand your professional nursing network, while making a difference to patient care by volunteering to facilitate unit, department, or hospital-wide initiatives.

Reflection Questions

- Describe your experience being involved in a project or committee? What did you learn?
- If you are not currently involved in any project or committee, what is stopping you from participating?

References

American Nurses Association. (2010). *Nursing professional development: Scope and standards of practice.* Silver Spring, MD: Author.

American Nurses Association. (2015). *ANA President Pamela F. Cipriano, PhD, RN, NEA-BC, FAAN, Responds to Comments on ABC's "The View"* [Press release]. Retrieved from http://www.nursingworld.org/FunctionalMenuCategories/MediaResources/PressReleases/ANA-President-Cipriano-Responds-to-Comments-on-ABCs-The-View.html

American Nurses Association. (2018). *About ANA.* Retrieved from https://www.nursingworld.org/ana/about-ana/

American Nurses Credentialing Center. (2019). *Magnet model—Creating a Magnet culture.* Retrieved from https://www.nursingworld.org/organizational-programs/magnet/magnet-model/

Clavelle, J., Porter-O'Grady, T., Weston, M., & Verran, J. A. (2016). Evolution of structural empowerment: Moving from shared to professional governance. *The Journal of Nursing Administration, 46*(6), 308–312. doi:10.1097/NNA.0000000000000350

Domrose, C. (2011). *Meeting Magnet: Creating committee participation is a challenge with big payoffs.* Retrieved from https://www.nurse.com/blog/2011/08/15/meeting-magnet-creating-committee-participation-is-a-challenge-with-big-payoffs/

Dyess, S. M., Opalinski, A., Saiswick, K., & Fox, V. (2016). Caring across the continuum, a call to nurse leaders to manifest values through action with community outreach. *Nursing Administration Quarterly, 40*(2), 137–145. doi:10.1097/NAQ.0000000000000157

Flaugher, M., Beyea, S. C., & Slattery, M. J. (2015). *Evidence-based practice made simple.* Brentwood, TN: HCPro.

Grigsby, R. K. (2008). *Committee, task force, team: What's the difference? Why does it matter?* Retrieved from https://www.aamc.org/download/164730/data/grigsby_committee_task_force_team.pdf

Matthews, J. (2012). Role of professional organizations in advocating for the nursing profession. *Online Journal of Issues in Nursing, 17*(1), 3. doi:10.3912/OJIN.Vol17No01Man03

Phillips, A. L., Nigro, O., Macolino, K. A., Scarborough, K. C., Doecke, C. J., Angley, M. T., & Shakib, S. (2014). Hospital admissions caused by adverse drug events: An Australian prospective study. *Australian Health Review, 38*(1), 51–57. doi:10.1071/AH12027

Porter-O'Grady, T., & Finnigan, S. (1984). *Shared governance for nursing: A creative approach to professional accountability.* Rockville, MD: Aspen Systems.

Schneider, A. (2015). *Nursing organizations: The role they play in professional development.* Retrieved from https://www.rn.com/nursing-organizations-the-role-they-play-in-professional-development/

Vanderbilt University Medical Center. (n.d.). *What is Shared Governance?* Retrieved from https://ww2.mc.vanderbilt.edu/Shared%20Governance/46398

Wilkins, C. (2018). The role of nurses in community outreach. *NEJM.* Retrieved from https://catalyst.nejm.org/videos/role-nurses-community-outreach/

Making a Difference in Research, Evidence-Based Practice, and Quality Improvement

Rhoda R. Redulla

"My classmate and I rewrote the paper and resubmitted it and the second time we submitted it, it was accepted. I thought the whole idea that you could publish your work was incredible and was instantly hooked."

—Carolyn Sun, PhD, RN, ANP-BC

Beginning with Florence Nightingale, research has been a part of the nursing profession for at least 200 years. The pledge to continuously improve practice prompts nurses to engage in research, evidence-based practice (EBP), and quality improvement (QI). Nurses use research to deliver care grounded on evidence that promotes quality health outcomes for individuals, families, communities, and healthcare systems. Research, EBP, and QI can be done in any setting: in the practice setting (ambulatory, acute, home care, community), academia, industry, and other areas where nurses practice.

Research seems to occur more frequently in the academic setting through the completion of requirements to fulfill an academic degree; for professors, this is integral to their scholarship or promotion for tenured status. In the practice environment, this may not happen so easily. This is contingent on the structures in place to support nurses to engage in research.

RESEARCH

The Nursing Research Process

The nursing research process involves identification of the research problem, determining the variables that will be measured, and the appropriate sample. This is followed by data collection, analysis, interpretation of data, and, finally, dissemination of findings.

One of the key skills that new nurses learn is to identify a clinical problem. Next, they identify the methodology on how to best address it and the remaining steps in the research process. In a nurse residency program, new nurses gain a deeper understanding on the differences between research, EBP, and QI. Nurses are also taught when to apply these methodologies. When there is no sufficient evidence to support a change or guide clinical practice, nurses explore the feasibility of doing a research study to generate evidence.

This chapter provides pointers to guide you on how to begin a research study, ideas on what resources are available, and other practical advice on how to conduct research. It is not intended to provide an in-depth instruction on the step-by-step nursing research process. Rather, it aims to inspire you to consider getting involved in research as you develop to your fullest potential as a nursing professional.

How to Identify Research Problems

Research problems evolve from questions that arise during encounters with patients, from gaps identified when performing a procedure, and from many other aspects of clinical practice. Constantly asking why, or questioning the implications of clinical decisions, often leads to ideas. In several research studies, the authors investigated the effectiveness of chewing gum in preventing postoperative ileus. A systematic review that followed stated that there is some evidence that chewing gum postoperatively may help recovery of gastrointestinal function by stimulating earlier resumption of bowel activity (Short et al., 2015). The article did not cover how this idea evolved. It could have been from a request by patients or a result of a healthcare team's discussion as they explored options to improve the quality of life and prevent complications for this patient population. This is a great example of how an idea evolved into a research study and generated new evidence to guide practice.

The National Institute of Nursing Research (NINR) is an entity within the U.S. National Institutes of Health that promotes and supports clinical and basic research to establish a scientific basis for the nursing care of individuals across the life span. The organization sets the priorities and agenda for nursing research (Box 5.1). The NINR Strategic Plan has set the following priorities:

- Symptom Science: Promoting Personalized Health Strategies
- Wellness: Promoting Health and Preventing Disease
- Self-Management: Improving Quality of Life for Individuals With Chronic Illness
- End-of-Life and Palliative Care: The Science of Compassion

BOX 5.1 TOPICS ENCOMPASSED BY THE NATIONAL INSTITUTE OF NURSING RESEARCH'S SCIENTIFIC PROGRAMS

- Exploring the mechanisms underlying symptoms of illness and developing personalized treatments that address these mechanisms through symptom science research
- Enhancing wellness by understanding the physical, behavioral, cultural, and environmental influences on health status and developing culturally tailored interventions to prevent illness and promote health
- Helping individuals with chronic conditions better understand and manage these conditions by engaging individuals as active participants in managing their own health
- Providing caregivers with better tools to fulfill their caregiving responsibilities and maintain their own quality of life
- Developing palliative care strategies to help individuals and families manage the symptoms of life-limiting conditions and plan for end-of-life decisions
- Using innovative technologies to develop novel interventions that deliver personalized care and real-time health information to patients, families, and health care providers
- Promoting the development of an innovative, multidisciplinary, and diverse nursing science workforce through a variety of training programs and mechanisms (NINR, 2016)

In a pediatric unit, a new nurse noted an opportunity on how the hospital is providing asthma education to the patients and their families. What is the best method? Is the reading level appropriate? When is the best time to provide the education? The nurse did an initial search in the literature but could only find a study that was done in the adult setting. Upon discussion with her manager, she was advised to meet with the nursing professional development specialist (or in some settings, known as the nurse educator). The nurse educator suggested that they reach out to the patient education committee. After receiving guidance from the patient education committee, the nurse met with the nurse researcher. The nurse researcher reviewed the research question, research design, and the next steps to prepare to seek approval from the institutional review board (IRB). The primary purpose of the IRB is to protect the rights and welfare of human subjects involved in research activities being conducted under its authority (www.irb.pitt.edu). In the absence of an IRB, the hospital may have an ethics committee that serves to perform similar duties of an IRB.

In a nonteaching hospital, there may be limited access to a nurse researcher. The hospital may then partner with another academic medical center or a nursing school. Doctorally prepared members of the faculty collaborate with nurses in the practice setting to conduct researches.

Research for New-to-Practice Nurses

Many new-to-practice nurses have access to a nurse residency program, which is intended to help new nurses transition to clinical practice. It also builds on the existing knowledge of nurses on research, EBP, and QI. The program typically runs for 6 to 12 months and develops critical thinking and clinical decision-making skills.

The Vizient/AACN (American Nurses Credentialing Program) Nurse Residency Program™ was established to support new graduate nurses as they transition into clinical practice. The program is designed to provide a structured environment for nurses to learn to:

- Use effective decision-making skills
- Provide clinical nursing leadership when administering care
- Incorporate research-based evidence into practice
- Strengthen their professional commitment to nursing
- Formulate an individual development plan

SUCCESS STORY

Stephanie O'Neill, BSN, RN

Senior Staff Nurse, Medical-Surgical/Transplant Unit, NewYork-Presbyterian/Weill Cornell Medical Center, New York

Stephanie successfully completed a nurse residency program and shared how the program has honed her EBP and research skills.

Tell us more about your current role and your journey in nursing so far.

When I was hired as a clinical nurse in 2017, little did I know that it was my life experiences that would be my driving force. My previous career choice of biomedical engineering drew me toward EBP and research. I am currently the co-chair of our nursing EBP/research council. My psychology background helped hone the skill sets required to be an active member and contributor to our nurse resident advisory board, co-chair of unit council, and recently a nursing board representative. These opportunities have afforded me the realization that my current role as a clinical nurse is not only about wearing the different hats for the patients and families, but about utilizing my most important hat of all, my "team hat." This, plus my involvement in EBP and research, puts me right at the forefront to do so.

How has the program helped you develop as a nurse? Also, specifically how has it developed your skills in research and EBP?

The biggest asset this program has added toward my professional development is my thinking cap. Always thinking, assessing, looking for ways to improve is what the nurse residency program has helped me develop as a new nurse. Through the program, I had the opportunity to learn firsthand from experts, including our program director, biomedical librarian, and nurse scientist. Our nurse scientist was committed to explain to me how to appraise the evidence and where to find evidence and use our library resources. Since I am in an environment driven to foster EBP and research, I had the great opportunity to attend some conferences such as "Symptom Science" and "How to Get Published." Through my training as a nurse resident, my interest to be involved in our EBP/Research Council was jumpstarted. At first, I thought the committee was intimidating, but with some guidance and a little nudging toward finding my confidence, I realized we are all NERDS, and it stuck as our team "nick name" (Nurses in EBP and Research Drive Science). With our recent Magnet® designation, the focus is no longer "How do we get there"; it's "How do we keep going?" EBP, QI, and research will help drive those answers! Our focus is also on how we continue to support each other in our "why" we are a nurse and to relentlessly work toward achieving favorable outcomes for our patients and their families.

What is your advice for new nurses?

A wise man once told me always to always "Be yourself."

What is your advice for new nurses?

In cliff note form, because sometimes that's all the time we have to read and easy to remember:

1. Always and forever ask questions. Never ever stop learning.
2. Never assume, but always assess! Know what you know. And "know/learn" what you do not know!
3. Be patient with yourself during your orientation, set goals, and take advantage of peer-to-peer review.
4. Closed-loop communication, and just communication in general is a must.
5. Always wear our vision, respect credo, and mission on your sleeves/heart, and never be afraid to be engaged.

Chapter 5 Making a Difference in Research, Evidence-Based Practice, and Quality Improvement

Research for Experienced Nurses

Experienced nurses have endless opportunities to engage in research. Highly motivated nurses move ahead with writing research proposals and requesting support from leaders to do so. For example, Cheryl, an advanced nurse clinician in the postsurgical unit, developed an interest in using aromatherapy to prevent nausea among postoperative patients. As a holistic nursing certified nurse, combined with her experience in caring for postsurgical patients, Cheryl was committed to improving care through research. During the annual goal setting process, she included "To conduct a research study using aromatherapy and other holistic methods" as one of her goals.

Other opportunities for experienced nurses to be involved in research:

- Fellowship Programs
- Involvement in professional organizations
- Applying for grants

Research for Nurse Leaders

Nurse leaders should be at the forefront of advancing a culture of inquiry and generating organizational support for research. The American Organization for Nursing Leadership (AONL) has identified a specific competency for nurse leaders to support this goal: emphasize utilization, dissemination, and participation in studies (AONL, 2015).

In one academic medical center, researchers examined the impact of the following structural interventions on nurses' use of library resources and nurses' knowledge, attitudes, and practices toward EBP (Carter, Rivera, Gallagher, & Cato, 2018):

> 1) EBP and research committee meetings, in which nurses were educated on how to formulate a clinical question and critically appraise a research article; 2) Academic Partners Program, in which nurse academicians provided scholarly mentorship and guidance during monthly committee meetings; 3) hiring of clinical nurse scientists who provided 1-on-1 education and mentorship to clinical nurses in EBP and research; and 4) a Nurse Residency Program partnership, in which newly graduated nurses were required to complete an EBP project. (p. 18)

These are some interventions that a nurse leader who is committed to foster a culture of inquiry can implement or at least advocate for.

SUCCESS STORY

Donna Zucker, PhD, RN, FAAN

Professor Emeritus, University of Massachusetts, Amherst

Dr. Donna Zucker is recognized as an expert in behavioral treatment for stress in incarcerated persons in the United States and abroad, particularly those incarcerated for substance misuse disorder. She is currently co-chair of the Eastern Nursing Research Society's Research Interest Group on Criminal Justice, Violence and Trauma; a member of the Board of the Academic Consortium on Criminal Justice Health; and a member of the University of Connecticut Center for Correctional Health Networks.

Dr. Zucker was the principal investigator on a Substance Abuse and Mental Health Services Administration (SAMHSA) grant (2016–2019), training up to 150 student nurses annually in screening, brief intervention, and referral to treatment. Additionally she is collaborating with forensic nurses from Saskatchewan, Canada, on tele-psych and psychiatric mental health nursing programs.

Dr. Zucker has developed several stress-reduction labyrinths for students, faculty, and incarcerated persons, adding to efforts across the community, campus, and school to increase civility. She is a Veriditas-certified labyrinth facilitator and has extensive training in mindfulness-based stress reduction and motivational interviewing.

What advice can you give to nurses who are new to research or interested to pursue research?

Clinical nurses without a doctoral degree should find a mentor, someone who is master's prepared, or an experienced nurse from the education department who has been published. For PhD students, the emphasis is on the last year of your coursework. You have to present your research and publish within the first 2 years of graduation. After my dissertation defense, my major professor had one clear message: that I have to publish within the next 2 years. Another piece of advice is for bachelor's- and master's-prepared nurses to be involved in their professional organizations. Membership can help you get connected to others in your areas of interest.

What was your first publication? How did you do it?

I got rejected the first time I submitted a manuscript. It was a findings paper from my dissertation. I even got rejected a couple more times. Then I went to a conference and met another attendee who was an online journal editor. I shared my work with her, and she asked me to send it to her (the online editor). And I got it published. That gave me the confidence to try again.

Why should nurses publish?

This may be a bit biased since I have worked in academia, but to be promoted within the organization, you need to publish at least 10 articles before you achieve tenure and then another 10 more to be promoted to professor. When I finished my PhD, research dissemination was a concept not necessarily translated quickly into practice. Sigma Theta Tau International, the honor society for nurses, prompted newer members like me of the importance of translating my work into practice. Publishing also demonstrates your currency in the field. My scholarly interest began with alcohol addiction; additionally I studied areas related to this phenomenon, including infection and chronic illness symptoms. I have done extensive work in corrections, mental health, and substance abuse. As I said, originally I focused on alcohol disease, which branched to the health issues of concern to the incarcerated population. This connected me with research being done in HIV, hepatitis C virus, and hepatitis B virus. During this work I became interested in the symptom of stress associated with incarcerated persons.

Who were your mentors?

In the early 2000s, I was hired along with three other faculty members on the tenure track. We created our own support system and established a peer mentorship group. We were committed to each other's development. In fact, we made this support group function in a structured way and went on to publish our experiences and outcomes. Here is an excerpt of the article published in the *Journal of Professional Nursing*:

> The peer research group is designed to help members develop
> programs of research that include internally and externally
> funded research, publication in peer-reviewed publications, and
> opportunities for doctoral students to work in the faculty member's
> program of research. . . . during meetings, members discuss their
> current scholarship, sharing successes and less-than-successful
> moments. We share reviewers' comments on our manuscripts and
> proposals so that we can all learn from our individual experiences.
> (Jacelon, Zucker, Henneman, & Stacciarini, 2003, p. 335)

What is your advice for nurses who are interested in research or would like to publish?

Seek out a mentor. Leverage skill through joining or creating a support group, and then get confident. My colleagues and I obtained two grants from my university to support peer mentoring. This supported research training, provided expert speakers, and created time away from campus to write and think. Today, many years later, I still have people asking me about peer mentoring, and the article we wrote together has been cited many times. Somehow, our group became expert in peer mentoring. I believe in paying it forward. My dean was very helpful to me, so I go the extra mile to be helpful to someone else. It is important to remember that you have not achieved your successes without the help of others. To reiterate, join a professional organization, research interest group, or clinical practice organization. This will expand your professional network tremendously.

EVIDENCE-BASED PRACTICE

How Nurses Can Make a Difference in EBP

EBP is the application of the best and current evidence. To provide the highest quality of care, nurses stay up to date on the most recent research findings and clinical guidelines. This they access through peer-reviewed journals and guidelines from professional organizations.

EBP 101

In nursing schools, EBP has been integrated into the curriculum. However, this is only applicable for recent nursing graduates. To fill the knowledge gap, some organizations have integrated EBP in the new nurse orientation program. The gap may still exist among experienced nurses. How can nurses become more familiar with EBP?

Participate in a Continuing Education Course

Inquire about course offerings from your education department. Check for research updates or educational programs offered within your institution or its partners.

Attend a Nursing Grand Rounds

Nursing grand rounds (NGR) showcase trends in healthcare, nursing practice, case studies, and other topics relevant to a broad group of nurses. I personally get invigorated and immediately think of ways to apply what I just learned after attending an NGR.

Attend a Nursing EBP or Research Symposium

This is another way to stay abreast on your EBP and research skills. Symposia are also great places to network.

Subscribe and Learn From Peer-Reviewed Nursing Journals

A peer-reviewed nursing journal features original research articles, evidence-based clinical applications, best practices, and QI reports.

HOW TO BE AN EVIDENCE-BASED PRACTITIONER

Do you think of yourself as an evidence-based practitioner? You become one by holding yourself accountable to improve the quality and safety of patients, support for patients' families, and enhance your practice environment.

Steps in EBP

ASSESS
- Assess the problem to determine pertinent issues.

ASK
- Using the PICO/T format, ask a clear, answerable question.

  P: Patient population

  I: Intervention

  C: Comparison intervention

  O: Outcome/s

ACQUIRE
- Search for evidence using healthcare databases (PubMed, CINAHL, PsychInfo, Cochrane).

APPRAISE
- Using critical appraisal tools, review and analyze the evidence.

APPLY
- Apply the evidence to your patients or setting.

SUCCESS STORY

Daphne Stannard, PhD, RN-BC, CNS, FCCM

Associate Professor, San Francisco State University School of Nursing, San Francisco; Visiting Professor, University of Adelaide, Australia

Tell us more about your current role and your professional journey in nursing. What are you most proud of?

After I completed my PhD in nursing, I set out for a career in academia and started as an assistant professor in nursing at San Francisco State University (SFSU). I loved the vibrant nature of the SFSU urban campus and the incredible diversity of the students and staff. But I also felt the tug to return to the service sector, as I greatly missed clinical practice. After receiving tenure and promotion, I returned to the University of California San Francisco (UCSF) Medical Center, where I had worked for many years in a variety of clinical roles while I was in graduate school. After several years working as the perianesthesia chief nurse specialist (CNS), I became the chief nurse researcher and founded the Institute for Nursing Excellence, which is a support department for nursing with three arms: clinical education, clinical inquiry, and clinical practice. In this role and as the Joanna Briggs Institute (JBI) Center director, I helped to establish the UCSF JBI Center for Evidence Synthesis and Implementation: A Joanna Briggs Center of Excellence and set up structures and processes whereby clinical nurses had the educational, research, and practice support they needed to consistently and reliably deliver excellent patient and family care. I am proud of that work, but I am also proud of the EBP mentoring and program development in which I have been involved over the years with students, clinical nurses, and international EBP fellows. To that end, I have returned to SFSU School of Nursing to continue my nursing research and EBP activities and to mentor undergraduate and graduate nursing students again.

What made you become interested in EBP and research?

I have always been interested in how and why things work the way they do, and I have an internal drive to improve and build structures and processes to ensure the highest quality outcomes. EBP is a natural fit for me because I am clinically oriented and enjoy thinking about how to improve any and all clinical issues. Sometimes, that question will lead to primary research and discovery, and as the former chief nurse researcher at UCSF, I welcomed that inquiry! But I also highly value QI work (also known as implementation), as that is when previously discovered solutions are applied to local settings and evaluated as to whether or not they helped to improve outcomes or make a difference.

What is your advice for beginning nurses as they attempt to integrate EBP/research in their day-to-day practice? Advice for experienced nurses?

For all nurses, EBP is an indispensable component of nursing practice and, I would argue, is actually woven into the nursing process. All that is needed to embrace EBP as part of one's daily practice is engagement with the clinical situation, clinical curiosity, and access to best available evidence. I encourage all nurses to get involved in professional and specialty organizations, as many offer journal clubs and other resources to assist a nurse at any stage of their career. For experienced nurses in particular, dive in! Get involved in local projects and mentor the junior nurses in your unit. You have much wisdom to share, and we all have much to learn!

How can leaders support EBP/research?

I am a firm believer that nursing practice will follow when the appropriate processes and structures are in place to support that practice. EBP comes naturally to most nurses, as they see clinical issues and can often readily think of good solutions. Nurse leaders need to help support and boost the curiosity, engagement, and active questioning that frontline staff have and look to marshal resources to assist with project work if necessary. Clinical nurse specialists, nursing professional development specialists, and clinical nurse researchers are great resources for staff if the facility has access to these disciplines, and if not, partnering with a local school of nursing is another solution to get programs and structures, such as EBP fellow programs and journal clubs, set up and running.

QUALITY IMPROVEMENT

Healthcare professionals, including nurses, can feel challenged and often lack training in QI methods, which makes it challenging to participate in improvement efforts (Silver et al., 2016). QI involves a collaborative effort between the healthcare team and stakeholders to systematically improve the ways care is delivered to patients. Nurses have demonstrated meaningful contributions when involved in QI projects. How can you be involved and make a difference in these projects? First, let's review the basics of QI.

Steps in QI

Identify the Problem or Issue

Is your hospital struggling with an issue about poor preparation of patients prior to a procedure? Or poor compliance with the time-out procedure? Are your patient experience scores on medication side effects? These are common problems that can be potentially addressed through a QI project. The first step in QI is to clearly identify the problem or issue you are trying to solve.

Enlist a Core Change Team

In a QI project, an interprofessional team is formed by first identifying the stakeholders involved in the issue. A stakeholder is someone who is impacted by or can contribute to an initiative or someone who can influence its success or failure (Brugha & Varvasovszky, 2000).

Stakeholders can include both individuals and organizations, internal or external to your organization such as caregivers, clinicians, advocacy groups, and policy makers.

A project team includes project lead, a project manager, process owners, clinicians and administrative staff, a quality coach, and a data analyst. Some other roles are created specific to the project or the organization. Many organizations have an executive sponsor, who is an individual with power and leadership skill within the organization who can be approached when needed to secure resources and remove barriers. Other organizations have patient family advisers in the team, who share their experience and unique perspective in the processes involved.

Here are some roles in a project team and examples of the functions associated with each role (IHI, n.d.).

Project Lead

- Oversee all aspects of the project
- Lead the team in developing project aims, methods, and measurement strategy
- Provide clinical expertise and perspective

Project Manager

- Develop and monitor project plan including deliverables, milestones, tasks, and timeline
- Plan, coordinate, facilitate, and document meetings and improvement activities, including but not limited to project team meetings, sponsor updates, advisory meetings, express workouts, training sessions, and so forth

Process Owners

- Ensure the process meets patient, clinician, and healthcare system needs
- Ensure clinicians and administrative staff are engaged in improvement activities that affect the process
- Ensure that improvements are incorporated into standard operating procedures and sustained

Clinicians and Administrative Staff

- Develop and participate in Plan-Do-Study-Act (PDSA) initiatives
- Champion improvement activities with other clinicians and staff (IHI, n.d.)

Nurses contribute to many aspects of QI. QI projects have nurse leaders as executive sponsors or process owners. Nurses in clinical roles are integral in implementing improvement activities by serving as champions of change. Participating in a QI initiative is a great opportunity for nurses to hone their leadership skills. See Table 5.1 for different types of improvement frameworks.

Table 5.1

	Lean	Six Sigma	Model for Improvement
Select an Improvement Framework			
Main Process/ Theme/ Approach	**Continuous improvement:** Achieved by distinguishing value-added activities from nonvalue-added activities (waste)	**DMAIC:** Define Measure Analyze Improve Control	**Asks three questions:** ■ What are we trying to accomplish? ■ How will we know that a change is an improvement? ■ What change can we do that will result in an improvement?
Main Tools	Japanese names of methods: Gemba Kaizen event PDSA	ANOVA Mathematical modeling Control charts	PDSA cycle Rapid cycle testing

ANOVA, analysis of variance; PDSA, Plan-Do-Study-Act.

Examples of How Nurses Are Involved in QI

a. Nurses in the endoscopy unit participate in a multidisciplinary initiative to reduce unnecessary waste in multidose medications.

b. Nurses in a cardiac unit initiated a project to reduce medication errors on the unit.

c. Wound care and ostomy nurses collaborated with the hospital quality team to reduce the hospital-acquired pressure injury rates.

THE 4Ps: PUBLICATION, POSTER, PODIUM, PODCAST

One of the most exciting aspects of successfully implementing a project is dissemination. Being able to share your work with colleagues and professionals within and outside the organization can bring you deep fulfillment and joy. It's a grand finale to any scholarly work. Do you remember the Hammerstein quote "A bell's not a bell 'til you ring it. A song's not a song 'til you sing it"? This quote resonates with me a lot when I think of project dissemination. It's also our ethical and professional obligation to share the work and have others learn from it. Beautiful, isn't it? Or you might be thinking, "Yes, but it's not that simple."

Many opportunities for scholarly dissemination are available to nurses. Various professional nursing organizations provide these opportunities at local, regional, national, and international meetings. Whether you are thinking of doing an oral presentation or submitting an abstract for a poster, you have many options.

Dissemination

A key step in any scholarly project is dissemination. Why disseminate? Imagine your team comes up with a novel population-specific tool, successfully implements it in your unit, keeps doing it, but did not have the opportunity to share it with the rest of the hospital or other hospitals that might benefit from your work. We have heard of prominent scientists who completed some of the most important breakthroughs in medicine or healthcare but never lived to see their work being implemented. Now, that may sound extreme to you. The point is that sharing your work with others who might benefit from it is important. Dissemination is included as a significant aspect in completing a project.

After completing a project, the project team proceeds to evaluate the work and explore opportunities for project dissemination, both internal and external.

Internal

You need not look far for internal dissemination of your work. This can occur within your unit's or department's monthly staff meeting. Arrange a good time with your supervisor. Be prepared to tailor the duration of your presentation according to the available time frame provided to you. If you implemented a project as part of an academic degree, most schools require that you present your project within your team, at the very least. This is aligned with the same viewpoint that sharing your scholarly work is a key step in accomplishing your project. For the capstone project I completed for my DNP at The Johns Hopkins University, I was required to present my project at our hospital. My project was the development and testing of a novel nurse-driven pathway in hepatitis C treatment, or more widely known as Project P.E.A.C.H.© (Pathway and Education towards Adherence and Completion in Hepatitis C management). I had to work within the time frame required by my academic program, and only had a few weeks to plan. I was lucky to be able to arrange a specific time that was feasible for most of the team members in our clinical division, including nurses, medical assistants, physicians, and the administrative support staff. After this initial session, I was requested by our nursing director to present at a larger audience during Nurses' Week. Other opportunities for me to disseminate my project also evolved from there.

Depending on the focus and scope of your project, you can look into sharing your work at other committee meetings, locally within your unit or department or hospital-wide.

Here are more examples:

- Two clinical nurses in a medical-surgical unit, Elizabeth and Emily, championed falls prevention on the unit and implemented a falls prevention safety bundle consisting of medication review during interdisciplinary rounds, hourly rounding, and door signs to communicate falls risks. After the first 3 months of implementation, the unit noted a decrease in the overall falls rate. Elizabeth and Emily presented their results at a 1:1 meeting with their manager, the monthly staff meeting, and then the divisional meeting known as "Medicine and Surgery Cluster Meeting." This meeting is a multidisciplinary meeting chaired by the physician lead on quality and safety. The following quarter, an annual call for posters at the hospital poster symposium was released. I'm sure you are thinking the two clinical nurses were most likely to submit an abstract. You are right. Elizabeth and Emily presented the falls prevention bundle initiative and shared their strategies and challenges to employees at the poster symposium.

- A nurse manager, Kaitlyn, along with two clinical nurses, Dorothy and Sean, developed a "Quick Wins" board, a communication tool that provides all members of the team a safe venue for proposing ideas and providing feedback for improvement. This project improved the unit's nursing engagement scores and, subsequently, the patient experience scores on nursing responsiveness. Initially, the manager and the team were invited to present at the hospital's nursing leadership council. Several other presentations at other meetings followed from there.

- At a pediatric ambulatory clinic, Carleen, a nurse practitioner, initiated a support group for children with diabetes. The support group and their parents meet once a month and receive guidance and support on various aspects of managing their disease. The hospital's Patient and Family Advisory Council (PFAC) learned about this work and wanted to acknowledge Carleen and her team's efforts to establish the support group. Carleen was invited to the PFAC meeting. The PFAC chair recognized Carleen and the pediatric ambulatory team and requested Carleen to present highlights of their work.

External

Many nurses aspire to present and share their scholarly work at a conference, whether local, regional, national, or even international.

When mentoring nurses, I get asked frequently, How do you find conferences to present? Start with conferences offered by organizations within your specialty. In my hospital, nurses from our oncology department submit abstracts to the Oncology Nurses Society Congress every year. Critical care nurses attend the National Teaching Institute (NTI) Conference offered by the American Association of Critical-Care Nurses (AACN). Many, if not all, professional nursing organizations send an annual call for abstracts to its members. Nonmembers learn about these opportunities directly through the nursing organization's website or other venues. In the example shared under internal presentations, Kaitlyn, the nurse manager, is a member of a professional organization and attends the annual conference. That year, the team submitted an abstract showcasing their work on the "Quick Wins" board. The abstract was accepted for podium presentation. Throughout the year, a huge range of QI, evidence implementation work, or original research is completed by nurses in various roles. Nurses also have numerous opportunities to share their work with an external audience.

How to Write an Abstract

Publication

Even experienced nurses may find writing an abstract off-putting. When you open the instructions for submission, it is easy to be discouraged seeing the multiple steps and detailed guidelines. Don't be. The instructions include many details to make both the submission and review processes easier for everyone.

Wood and Morrison (2011) shared some tips. When submitting, it is critical to choose the right meeting. Ask yourself:

- Will the audience be interested?
- Is there a theme to the meeting, and does my project/case fit with that theme?
- Has my mentor or another colleague attended/presented at the meeting? What is his or her advice?
- Where will the information have the most impact?
- Which meeting will provide the best networking opportunities?

Example of a "Call for Abstracts"

This section provides an overview of the submission requirements and guidelines. Here is an example of a "Call for Abstracts" from the American Nurses Credentialing Center (ANCC) Pathway to Excellence Program. Notice the judging criteria and the educational tracks offered. Pay attention to key dates.

Dates for Submission

Submissions will be accepted beginning Friday, June 2, 20XX. The deadline for abstract submissions is 11:59 pm Eastern on Monday, July 24, 20XX.

Notification

Accepted poster and concurrent podium session presenters will be notified in October 20XX. If you do not receive notification of acceptance or rejection for your abstract by October 2, 20XX, please send an email inquiry to conference staff at pteconabstract@ana.org.

Judging Criteria

Abstracts will be considered based on how well they fulfill the learning outcomes of the ANCC Pathway to Excellence Conference˚. All selections are made based on merit, with additional consideration given to those from Pathway to Excellence˚ or Pathway to Excellence in Long Term Care˚ organizations. There is no limit to the number of abstracts that may be submitted by a person or organization.

Learning Outcomes

Examine shared governance models and high-impact leadership strategies that cultivate nursing excellence and interprofessional partnership.

Evaluate evidence-based quality improvement initiatives for integration into the delivery of safe, effective patient care across all practice environments.

Assess methods of safeguarding the well-being of staff and the community to foster a culture of health.

Recognize the positive impact of lifelong learning on staff engagement and empowerment.

Educational Tracks

Shared Decision-Making & Leadership
    Safety & Quality
    Well-Being
    Professional Development

Who May Submit?

Those employed by a Pathway˚-designated organization at the time of submission.

    or

Researchers or educators working in partnership with a Pathway organization.

    or

Abstract submissions in support of the Pathway to Excellence˚ and Pathway to Excellence Long Term Care˚ standards who are not part of a Pathway to Excellence˚ organization

Submissions may not be from groups or persons with commercial interests.

For a research or QI abstract, it should include:

- Background and significance of the study/initiative
- Aims of the study/initiative
- Methods
- Results
- Discussion and implications

For an EBP project, you will see the PICO (Population, Intervention, Comparison Intervention, Outcomes) question included.

Poster

Poster presentations are a popular medium to disseminate best practice, innovation, and research studies in professional nursing conferences (Exhibit 5.1). Many posters, sometimes over a hundred, are displayed in a large hall. Poster-viewing sessions are integrated into the schedule. Conference participants review posters, ask questions from presenters, and identify best practices and solutions that they can take back to their teams. If you have not presented a poster before, I'm sure you are thinking, Where do I start?

Be Involved in a Project or Start One

Two examples were presented earlier: Kaitlyn and her team working on the "Quick Wins" board and Carleen on the support group for children with diabetes. These can be presented as posters. The poster, in an abbreviated format, is your work from its inception to completion and includes evaluation.

Kellianne and Christina's Experience

Kellianne and Christina, registered nurses in a Post Anesthesia Care Unit (PACU), were concerned about the noise level on the unit at night. Some patients were already struggling to have a restful sleep due to pain and discomfort. Others had a long and tedious day of treatments and tests. Kellianne and Christina committed to initiating a project to address this issue and promote a healing environment for the patients on their unit. They made a proposal to the nurse manager and the unit council during a monthly meeting. At that meeting, the nurse manager reviewed the patient satisfaction scores and highlighted how the ratings on the quietness of the hospital need improvement. Kellianne and Christina created a quietness-at-night plan with two other members of their team. The team reviewed the literature and noted "tuck-in" rounds as a best practice adopted by some hospitals. That year, Kellianne and Christina submitted their poster for presentation at the annual hospital poster symposium. Yearly, the PACU participates at the American Society of Perianesthesia Nurses (ASPAN) conference.

Reflect on Your Successful Outcomes

What has your department achieved in the past year? What changes in workflow or procedures have been made? Reflect on the impact of these changes and your contributions. These are all prompts for submitting a scholarly abstract.

Disseminate Your Work Internally Within Your Team

Presenting your work within your team is usually a safe space to obtain honest feedback regarding your work. This gives you an opportunity to make revisions before submitting to a larger body.

Here are examples of objectives for a poster session from the National Teaching Institute (NTI; AACN, 2019).

■ Identify best practices and solutions to advocate for patients across the continuum.
■ Identify areas within your own practice that may be impacted by nursing research.
■ Foster nursing research within your work environments to advance patient care and our profession.

Now, you are ready to make your poster.

Moyo (2019) shared some tips in creating a poster.

Compliant

■ It is your responsibility as a presenter to read and be **compliant**. with conference poster guidelines sent to you after your abstract is accepted for presentation.
■ Some organizations require either paper, digital, or both formats.

Catchy

■ Come up with a catchy title for your poster.
■ The title can be a question, a descriptor of the scope of work, or key findings.
■ Make it short and sharp like a hook!
■ Some organizations set a word count specifically for the title.

For the project I initiated—to create and test a nurse-driven pathway in hepatitis C—I coined an acronym to make it catchy: Project P.E.A.C.H. stands for Pathway, Education towards Adherence and Completion in Hepatitis C.

Clear

■ Your poster should "stand-alone" and readers should be able to easily understand your viewpoint without you being present to explain. (Organizations most often require you to be present. However, you serve as a complement to your poster, answering any questions.)

- The poster must have a clear, logical sequence.
- Check on visual clarity:
  - Title must be legible from 15 to 20 feet and body from 4 to 6 feet.
  - Darker text over light background is better; avoid "shadow" effect in text.

Concise

- Be clear and succinct. Bullet points are ideal.
- A wordy, busy poster may discourage attendees from reading your poster.
- Use pictures and graphics.

Clutter-Free

- Carefully consider the amount of text, font size, and font type.
- Choose fonts that are easy to read: sans serif for title/subtitle (Tahoma); serif for body (Times New Roman).
- Do not mix font types in the body of text.

Exhibit 5.1   Example of a Poster Template

OPERATION: SHHH! REDUCING NOISE IN THE PACU

Team Leaders: Kellianne Morgan, BSN, RN & Christina Stigliano, BSN, RN

NewYork-Presbyterian/Weill Cornell Medical Center

Background

- At NewYork-Presbyterian/Weill Cornell Medical Center, Post Anesthesia Care Unit (PACU), bed requests from Ambulatory Surgery F10 Operating Room (OR) to the F10 PACU were made through phone calls.
- These phone calls from the OR resulted in a high volume of noise in the PACU.
- The American Society of PeriAnesthesia Nurses (ASPAN, 2017) Standard II Environment of Care states that "perianesthesia nursing practice promotes and maintains a safe, comfortable and therapeutic environment."
- PICO: Will the combined utilization of technology and daily quiet hours create a more calming environment in the PACU?

Methods

- In July 2017, an electronic notification of bed requests called the Electronic Call Back (ECB) from the OR to the PACU was created.
- Interdisciplinary education took place for the staff in the OR and PACU regarding utilization of technology, including Mobile Heartbeat and the new ECB.
- During quiet hours, lights are dimmed, and staff members speak in a quiet and calming voice. A "noise champion" is assigned daily to introduce the quiet hours.
- IRB approval was not required for this performance improvement project.

NOTE: Some details of the poster were modified for demonstration purposes.

Results

- With the implementation of ECB, the volume of phone calls decreased significantly one month after the implementation of the project.
- The decrease in the volume of phone calls also resulted in a decrease in noise.
- A unit-wide survey was performed to obtain feedback on the modifications made on the unit.
- 100% of Registered Nurses (RNs) are satisfied with the new ECB and quiet hours.
- 92% of employees reported that during quiet hours, they speak in a softer tone to create a quiet and more therapeutic environment.

Chart Title

Discussion

- Evidence supports that a noisy environment can alter the patients' healing process and impair recovery.
- By implementing noise reduction techniques such as decreasing the frequency of phone call interruptions and quiet hours, the PACU can promote an optimal healing environment for patients recovering from surgery.
- Further efforts will include the implementation of white noise machines, aromatherapy, and continued use of technology.

References

American Society of PeriAnesthesia Nurses. 2016–2017 Standards of Perianesthesiology Nursing Practice. The American Society of PeriAnesthesia Nurses, Cherry Hill, NJ 2006.

Raymond, S. Goss, J. Leach, E. Latham, K. Pegram, M. Sullivan, C. Steele, R. & Cunningham, E. (2011) Professional Awareness concerning unnecessary noise in the PACU. Journal of PeriAnesthesia Nursing, 26(3), 194.

For more information, please contact: (NAME, TITLE) at CONTACT INFO. (WORK Email and /or Phone number).

IRB, institutional review board.

Source: **Courtesy of Kellianne Morgan and Christina Stigliano.**

Podium

You submitted an abstract, checked "either oral or poster," and just got notified that your submission was accepted for a podium presentation. What a great way to cap all your hard work on your project. If this will be your first time, you can expect to feel more nervous than excited initially. Even pros get the jitters before a presentation. With appropriate planning and preparation, you will shine.

Mai, Minehart, and Pian-Smith (2019) published seven tips for an engaging and memorable presentation. I added my own ideas and experience to each.

Tip 1: Know Your Audience: Before and During Your Talk

Through my previous experience as a nurse educator, I came across an online audience response system (ARS) called "Poll Everywhere" allowing participants to use their own mobile phones. Before this technology, we used automated clickers, which are distributed to the audience. I would integrate audience polling questions throughout the presentation but would take the opportunity in the beginning to use it to get to know my audience. Knowing your audience goes a long way on how you can successfully connect with them.

For my presentation on EBP, these were my polling questions:

I am confident in implementing an EBP project.

a. Strongly agree
b. Agree
c. Neither agree nor disagree
d. Disagree
e. Strongly disagree

When I presented on the nursing management of hepatitis C, I used Patricia Benner's model. I asked participants to identify their level of experience:

a. Novice
b. Advanced beginner
c. Competent
d. Proficient
e. Expert

For my hepatitis C presentation, I learned that the majority of participants considered themselves a novice on the topic. There were a few in the advanced beginner and proficient categories. Knowing this at the start of my talk, I focused on the information for the novice audience and engaged the advanced beginner and proficient nurses to share their experience.

Tip 2: Tell a Story

Stories connect people (Mai et al., 2019). Tell a story about one of your patients, your team, or anything that conveys how the topic is important to you. In one of my talks, I shared a story about one of my patients who will always remind me to look past an initial impression of a patient or family. This example evoked a lot of discussion from the audience, including empathy in the healthcare profession.

Tip 3: Trigger Videos

Trigger videos are short clips, either from a public source or your own, that relates to your topic. After showing the video, be prepared with a debriefing or a few discussion questions.

Tip 4: Think–Pair–Share

In this technique, participants first reflect quietly about the idea, then pair with neighbors to discuss, and then share to the bigger audience. Another way to do this is to divide the audience in small groups (more than a pair) and then do a large group discussion.

Tip 5: Role Play

I find role plays to be an effective way for learners to apply content in a real-world context. To plan the role play, the group brainstorms on scenarios and roles. They simulate several possibilities and outcomes of the topic presented, then decide on their final presentation.

Tip 6: "Flip the Classroom"

"Flipping the classroom" means having learners prepare before the teaching session. In a conference setting, this may not be feasible all the time, but it can be done. It may work better for a smaller audience where participants are preregistered. You can have the organizer send the materials to the participants.

Tip 7: Applying the "Take-Home Message"

Challenge the participants with a change in their behavior as a result of what they just learned.

Publication

How to Publish Your Article

I can't tell you how many nurses I have met who would say, "You can let me do anything. Just don't let me write." Nantz and Britt (2015, p. 42) could have not said it more perfectly: "Most nurses focus on honing their clinical skills, not on polishing their writing skills." Publishing your work is one huge step for you to be viewed as an expert. So, why not invest more time and effort to develop it?

Here are some steps to get you started.

1. *Decide on a topic. Write about what you are passionate about. This makes it easier. One of the first peer-reviewed articles I have wrote was on physician–patient communication. I was a clinical nurse working in the gastroenterology and hepatology clinic. Every day, I would witness a challenging conversation between one of our physicians and a patient or family member. Countless times, I saw conversations regarding a terminal diagnosis, or failed treatment of a chronic disease, and several other tough scenarios. I also saw many conversations where I thought, with more deliberate intention, the communication could have been 101% better. This spurred my interest to read more on the topic and I later found myself writing a literature review. I took this a step further and went on to write a feature article on the topic. You can do the same thing. Write about your interest or expertise. In the case of disseminating your scholarly work, this first step is already done for you. You have a topic.*

2. *Do a preliminary research on the topic.* Search for articles on the topic you've selected to write about to find out if a gap exists in the current literature. Look out for "call for articles." A few times a year, some journals release a list of topics they are interested to publish.

3. Write a letter of inquiry. Check the journal's author's page. Some journals post a template and ask for specific information for you to include when submitting your query.

4. *Develop your outline and start writing your first draft.* Now, you are ready to submit your article. A quick but important tip: Once you hit the "submit" button, get into the mind-set that this is just the beginning of the editing aspect of your work. Expect to obtain comments and requests for revision. The outcome of your initial submission could either be (a) accepted with minor revisions, (b) accepted with major revisions, or (c) rejected.

5. *Acceptance of your article.* After your article is submitted for publication, expect to receive a checklist of remaining tasks from the editor-in-chief or the production editor. This may include signing a copyright release form, clarifying references, confirming your institutional affiliation, and other minor work.

Podcast

With the increasing rage over podcasts in recent years, you have most likely tuned in to one. A podcast is an audio file that a user can download to a personal device (tablet, phone, or computer) for easy listening (Wikipedia, 2020). A podcast features a host who talks on a topic. The discussion can be either totally spontaneous or scripted and structured. You can be motivated to initiate your podcast for a variety of reasons: share your passion on a topic, advocate for your interest, increase professional visibility, and engage a network of influencers. Not to forget, it can be a valuable platform for dissemination of your scholarly work. Yes, the 4th P in publication, podium, poster, and … podcast! You can transform your presentation slides or poster into a podcast.

Ekta Vohra, BSN, RN, CWON, was featured in WOC Talk, a podcast presented by the Wound, Ostomy and Continence Nurses Society™. Ekta presented her organization's journey in meeting the demand of a 257% increase in ostomy patient visits and 138% in wound patient visits. Ekta and the team at her institution worked to research and measure the demand they were facing and understand the cost savings associated with adding additional full-time staff to meet this demand (WOC Talk, 2020). This is a great example of how a quality improvement project can be shared via a podcast. You can access the podcast here: https://woctalk.simplecast.com/episodes/meeting-the-demand-how-one-department-increased-their-woc-nurse-workforce-ep37-H8LRsrfE.

SUCCESS STORY

Carolyn Sun, PhD, RN, ANP-BC

Assistant Professor, Hunter College, New York City
Nurse Researcher/Nurse Scientist, NewYork-Presbyterian Hospital, New York City

Describe your professional nursing journey, including your current role.

I started out as a graphic designer but quickly felt like I wanted a job with a more altruistic aspect, so I went back to school for nursing. I took a job as a nurse working on an inpatient orthopedic and oncology floor at the University of Washington. I later went on to work in an outpatient chemo clinic at University of California, Los Angeles (UCLA), med/surg at University of California, San Francisco (UCSF), and a student health clinic in San Francisco before going back to school for my adult nurse practitioner degree at New York University (NYU). I then worked as an adult nurse practitioner in the NBC Universal employee health clinic while working on my PhD at the Columbia University School of Nursing (CUSON). After graduating, I held a 1-year postdoctoral position in the Office of Global Initiatives at CUSON, working on global health nursing research, before being hired in my current position as a jointly appointed nurse researcher between CUSON and NewYork-Presbyterian (NYP).

Describe your experience with your first scholarly presentation and publication. How did these opportunities come up?

My first publication was during my masters program at NYU. I had done a scholarly project with classmates, and we decided to try to get it published under the guidance of our adviser, Caroline Dorsen. I think we were actually rejected, but because I didn't know what I was doing, I took the letter as an opportunity to improve the paper. My classmate and I rewrote the paper and resubmitted it, and the second time we submitted it, it was accepted. I thought the whole idea that you could publish your work was incredible and was instantly hooked.

My first presentation came much later and was at the Eastern Nursing Research Society annual conference. My adviser, Elaine Larson, encouraged me to submit with a team of other researchers on our global health work. She helped me prepare and reviewed my slides. Columbia School of Nursing also has a forum to practice talks with other colleagues, which I participated in. Even though I was presenting work that was already published, I was incredibly nervous, and I couldn't get my slides up—a friend helped me get them up at the last second. I think I practiced more for that presentation than for my dissertation defense (to be fair, a lot of what I presented went into my dissertation presentation). In the end, everything went very well, but it reinforced an important lesson: We can't be successful without the help of our colleagues.

What are one or two pieces of advice that you can share for nurses who are considering to publish or present?

First of all, don't give up—I think persistence is 90% of success. The other 10% has to do with the quality of the writing and research. Second, don't be afraid to ask for help—we all have to help each other, and we've all been in the position where we need help. It is very rare to publish as a sole author (and I think increasingly frowned upon—we need to show our collaboration with others). Ask others to review and edit your work; if they make a substantial contribution, don't hesitate to add them as author. You can ask other nurses, but reaching out across disciplines can be a good idea as well—other professionals can contribute and expand our work to be more generalizable and applicable in other fields. This is true from the beginning when you're planning your study but is also true through the writing and publication process. Finally, early on, spend some time carefully selecting the target journal. Besides helping you craft your paper to meet the journal's guidelines, picking a journal that has an audience interested in your study will improve the likelihood of acceptance and save you a lot of time and trouble in the long run.

What are you most proud of, professionally?

I am most proud of the position I hold as a jointly appointed researcher between two of the world's finest institutions (referring to her immediate past organizations). Not only do I get to work with one of the greatest academic institutions and top nursing schools in the world (Columbia University School of Nursing), I get to work in one of the nation's finest and certainly the nation's top five hospitals (NewYork-Presbyterian). This allows me to collaborate with nurses on the ground; this sounds like an obvious thing to do, but unfortunately, there remains a gap between the clinic and academic. I truly believe that improving nursing practice is key to improving patient outcomes, and I hope that my efforts will have a substantial and lasting impact on health outcomes. I am proud to be building a bridge between clinical and academic silos to improve the evidence base for nurses, and subsequently patient outcomes, both locally and globally.

I have also had the pleasure of working with nurses, nurse faculty, and nurse scientists all over the world to improve nursing practice and patient outcomes through my research. Finally, I now am working at Hunter-Bellevue School of Nursing. Hunter is part of the City University of New York, which was founded with the purpose to promote the upward mobility of the disadvantaged. I am proud to be a part of such an honorable effort and really see that this is being done when I look at the diversity of students and the adversities they've overcome to achieve their dreams and become part of the nursing workforce. I truly believe that improving nursing practice is key to improving patient outcomes. I hope that my efforts will have a substantial and sustained impact on health outcomes for everyone everywhere.

THE BOTTOM LINE

You will see how being part of an initiative or leading a project can take you on a very rewarding journey of professional advancement and scholarship. An expectation after completing a scholarly project is to share how you did it, your findings, and overall experience. I would be the first advocate of "Start with the end in mind" (read: Start with a dissemination plan in mind). Don't forget to include this in your project plan. Also, if you have recently completed a poster, you almost have a first draft of a manuscript done. Well, that's the positive approach. Realistically speaking, writing a manuscript involves a lot of work and commitment. However, having bullet points of the background, methodology, findings, and implications for practice in a poster captures the same major elements typically required in an article. Hicks (2015) pointed out that the overlap between a podium or poster presentation and a fully developed manuscript is quite significant; the difference is in the style of presentation.

References

American Association of Critical-Care Nurses. (2019). Research Poster Sessions, National Teaching Institute. Retrieved from https://www.aacn .org/conferences-and-events/events-calendar/national-events/event

-sessions/national-teaching-institute---2019/pos115/research-poster -presentations

American Organization for Nurse Leaders. (2015). *Nurse manager competencies.* Retrieved from https://www.aonl.org/system/files/media/file/ 2019/06/nurse-manager-competencies.pdf

Brugha, R., & Varvasovszky, Z. (2000). Stakeholder analysis: A review. *Health Policy Plan, 15*(3), 239–246. doi:10.1093/heapol/15.3.239

Carter, E. J., Rivera, R. R., Gallagher, K. A., & Cato, K. D. (2018). Targeted interventions to advance a culture of inquiry at a large, multi-campus hospital among nurses. *Journal of Nursing Administration, 48*(1), 18–24. doi:10.1097/NNA.0000000000000565

Hicks, R. R. (2015). Transforming a presentation to a publication: Tips for nurse practitioners. Journal of the American *Association of Nurse Practitioners, 27*(9), 488–496. doi:10.1002/2327-6924.12228

Institute for Healthcare Improvement. (n.d.). *Improvement team roles & responsibilities.* Retrieved from http://app.ihi.org/FacultyDocuments/ Events/Event-2930/Presentation-16185/Document-13111/Presentation _Improvement_Team_Roles_and_Responsibilities.pdf

Jacelon, C. S., Zucker, D. M., Staccarini, J., & Henneman, E. A. (2003). Peer mentoring for tenure track faculty. *Journal of Professional Nursing, 19*(6), 335–338. doi:10.1016/S8755-7223(03)00131-5

Mai, C. L., Minehart, R. D., & Pian-Smith, M. C. (2019). Seven tips for giving an engaging and memorable presentation. *BJA Education, 19*(9), 274–275. doi:10.1016/j.bjae.2019.05.002

Moyo, M. (2019). The 5Cs for developing an effective poster presentation. *Journal of Radiology Nursing, 38*(3), 210–212. doi:10.1016/j. jradnu.2019.05.015

Nantz, S., & Britt, S. (2015). How to get your article published. *American Nurse Today.* Retrieved from https://www.myamericannurse.com/wp -content/uploads/2015/09/ant9-Writing-820.pdf

National Institute of Nursing Research. (2016). *NINR strategic plan: "Advancing science, improving lives."* Retrieved from https://www.ninr .nih.gov/newsandinformation/publications/strategic-plan

Short, V., Herbert, G., Perry, R., Atkinson, C., Ness, A. R., Penfold, C., . . . Lewis, S. J. (2015). Chewing gum for postoperative recovery of gastrointestinal function. *Cochrane Database of Systematic Reviews, 2,* CD006506. doi:10.1002/14651858.CD006506.pub3

Silver, S. A., Harel, Z., McQuillan, R., Weizman, A. V., Thomas, A., Chertow, G. M., . . . Chan, C. T. (2016). How to begin a quality improvement project. *Clinical Journal of the American Society of Nephrology, 11*(5), 893–900. doi:10.2215/CJN.11491015

Wikipedia. (2020). *Podcasts.* Retrieved from https://en.wikipedia.org/wiki/ Podcast

WOC Talk. (2020). *Meeting the demand: How one department increased their WOC nurse workforce.* Retrieved from https://woctalk.simplecast.com/ episodes/meeting-the-demand-how-one-department-increased-their -woc-nurse-workforce-ep37-H8LRsrfE

Wood, G. J., & Morrison, R. S. (2011) Writing abstracts and posters for national meetings. *Journal of Palliative Medicine, 14*(3), 353–359. doi:10.1089/jpm.2010.0171

Seeking Your Mentor

Patricia Toth

"A mentor is someone who allows you to see the hope inside yourself."
—Oprah Winfrey (Everwise, 2015)

In this chapter, we discuss mentors: who they are, why you need one, preceptor versus mentor, and how you can be a mentor. Terms such as *mentor* and *preceptor* are frequently used interchangeably. The terms *coach* and *facilitator* are sometimes used as well. Their meanings vary slightly, but the need for a mentor and/or preceptor is ever present in nursing. At every stage of your career, you may realize that you would benefit from interaction with an experienced nurse with your best interest at heart. Seeking a mentor is a sign of your ambition, confidence, and readiness for growth and development. I have had the privilege of having a few mentors and being a mentor throughout my career. I have found a mentor to be a wonderful asset as you consider advancing in or making changes within your career.

WHAT IS A MENTOR?

We acquired the word *mentor* from the literature of ancient Greece. In Homer's epic *The Odyssey*, Odysseus was away from home, fighting and journeying for 20 years. During that time, Telemachus, the son he left as a babe in arms, grew up under the supervision of Mentor, an old and trusted friend. When the goddess Athena decided it was time to complete the education of young Telemachus, she visited him, disguised as Mentor, and they set out together to learn about his father. Today, we use the word *mentor* for anyone who is a positive, guiding influence in another (usually younger) person's life (Merriam-Webster .com, n.d.). Dictionary.com (n.d.) states that a mentor is a wise or trusted counselor or teacher and influential senior sponsor or supporter.

A mentor is someone who provides invaluable advice, perspective, and guidance as you begin your career or advance in it. In nursing, there are so many opportunities for advancement, specialization, and career paths to pursue that a mentor can help in identifying and achieving your career goals. A mentor can be a coach, role model, counselor, and resource. The relationship can be formal or informal and may change as the needs of the mentee evolve. A mentor listens, inspires, motivates, offers guidance, discusses goals, and offers support. A mentor could introduce you to contacts who could assist in furthering your career. Hnatiuk (2013) succinctly puts this topic into focus when she wrote that you may be a newly graduated nurse or an experienced nurse taking a new position; if you need some guidance in your career, a mentor could assist you with your decisions. Rolfe (2017) lists the following as qualities of a mentor:

- Communication skills
- Being a sounding board
- Giving guidance
- Providing feedback
- Time and willingness to contribute
- Confidentiality (p. 41)

A mentoring relationship can be formed at any point in your career. A mentor recognizes and encourages potential. "Successful mentoring relationships are built on trust, openness to self-disclosure, affirmation and willingness, and skill in giving and receiving feedback" (Hnatiuk, 2013, p. 3). Someone whom I consider to be a mentor listened intently as I discussed the possibility of going to school for my DNP. She always said that I should just think it through and pursue what was best for me. During another discussion about going to school, she actually never said a word, and her silence made me talk more. I kept talking until I had an entire and complete pro/con list that I had not been able to verbalize before. When I read my list, I could not find a compelling reason not to go to school. As I let out a sigh of relief, she broke her silence and said, "It's about time!" I needed to completely think it through from all aspects before deciding, and she knew me well enough to make me take my time and decide.

Every nurse does not have to be a formal mentor to pay it forward and have an influence on a nurse, especially one who is new to your unit. As an experienced nurse, reach out and check in with any new nurses on your unit. Ask them how they are doing and if they have any questions. The new nurse will appreciate it and may look to you as a mentor or friend in the future.

MENTORING IN THE PRACTICE SETTING

The American Nurses Credentialing Center (ANCC) Magnet Recognition Program' recognizes the value of mentoring. One of the standards under the transformational leadership domain requires organizations to demonstrate mentoring activities of nurses at all levels—clinical nurses, advanced practice nurses, nurse managers, and nurse directors—including the chief nursing officer (CNO). Magnet'-recognized organizations align their leadership development programs with this framework.

Stanford Health Care (SHC), a Magnet organization, started its mentoring program in 2004 and was created to help new graduate nurses succeed in their first nursing positions. The program has evolved since its inception and now includes nurse residents, experienced nurses new to SHC, and nurses moving to other units within SHC (Stanford Health Care Mentoring Program, 2019).

Nurses who have completed the program shared their reflection. Here is one of the testimonials.

> *"Being mentored really put me right into being on a unit after my new grad program here at Stanford. There was a formal educational process which was really helpful—papers to read and discuss, things to think about as I went about the real work of being a nurse. I also met my mentor off-site, at coffee shops and was able to get valuable knowledge and support in a calm place where we could really focus on the conversation. The mentoring really helped me get into the routine of the unit very quickly and feel comfortable."*
>
> —Chelsea Simkins, RN, Mentee

MENTORING IN NURSING EDUCATION

Nurses new to practice or new to their unit do not exclusively benefit from mentorship. Shaikh (2017) discusses the benefits of a mentor to someone new to nursing education both in the hospital or in a university setting. Mentorship in nursing education leads to job satisfaction and improved teaching skills and team building. A successful mentor for those in nursing education, according to Shaikh (2017), has several roles:

- Provide professional support: This could include offering academic survival skills, helping with writing skills, and starting the new educator with introductions and networking.

- Feedback and evaluation: Mentors provide feedback on any or all aspects of the new educator's development.
- Psychosocial support: Mentors offer support during stressful times for the mentee.
- Role modeling: Mentors can shape ideas, instill confidence, and empower the mentee.
- Ethics: Mentees may experience different types of ethical dilemmas in education than as a staff nurse. Mentors can give them the tools to help them address these situations.
- Research and academia: The mentor should encourage scientific inquiry so the mentee can experience research and publication.

The mentoring relationship depends upon effective communication and interactions among all stakeholders. Nursing education, within the hospital or in the university, is a different type of nursing. As a former clinical instructor in a university and former professional development specialist in a hospital, I know that you need to be confident in your patient care skills as well as your interpersonal skills to be successful in either area. As a university professor or clinical instructor, you need to learn to teach to several students. Your confidence is tested from all sides; you never know which question is going to stump you. In the hospital, the nurse educator can have several jobs; they can be a project manager or just responsible for the education of a specific unit. All of this is new to someone joining nursing education. A mentor can guide you through learning to expand evidence-based practice as a faculty researcher to help move the profession forward. Your mentor can assist you in navigating moral and ethical issues that may arise in education. After you master your education position, you and your mentor can discuss how to advance your new career.

MENTORING IN NURSING LEADERSHIP

A nursing leader needs to achieve success at the individual and organizational level, according to Montavio and Veenema (2015). Mentorship is not thoroughly engrained in nursing as a profession. The gap is very evident in the realm of nursing leadership. Future nurse leaders need to develop knowledge in political and cultural savvy for the entire hospital or health system, not just one unit. Nursing leaders need to develop health policy and be part of creating a better system of care. New leaders are not accustomed to creating policies that affect staff on a global level; they are used to care plans for a specific patient. Mentoring in nursing leadership can be simply classified as leaders mentoring leaders. Your mentor, as you become a new leader, can help you learn coaching techniques and how to develop and manage your high-performing teams. Everything is new in the world of leadership, and a mentor will help you navigate your way through.

WHY DO YOU NEED A MENTOR?

A mentoring relationship can give you an edge in a competitive market. Wouldn't you benefit from the guidance and experience of someone who can help you navigate the early part of your career and possibly open doors for you in the later portion of your career?

Nursing is not the only profession that suggests that new staff need a mentor. Businesses use mentors to share their experiences on leadership, business skills, and more. Steve Jobs, former CEO of Apple, mentored Kelli Richards by guiding her through her MBA and bolstered her self-confidence to leave Apple and go out on her own to become CEO of the All Access group (Everwise, 2015).

A mentor can help shorten your learning curve and increase your self-confidence, and can provide you with many advantages. A mentor can introduce you to new possibilities and help you to identify new opportunities. Mentors are cheerleaders, open and honest, and accessible. They can positively influence a nurse's personal and professional growth. One reason that I have sought mentors is so they can help me to plan and guide my career trajectory. I remember a mentor discussing the politics of the hospital and what might be the best way to navigate through to advance my career. That "insider information" was valuable to me at that time and opened my mind to new ideas.

BENEFITS OF MENTORSHIP IN NURSING

Mentoring is a powerful personal and career development tool that can enable the mentee to achieve their life's goals and aspirations. Nursing, as a profession, is unique. Our knowledge aligns with our physician counterparts and is based on evidence, which is ever growing. We learn anatomy and physiology to understand what we are assessing, chemistry to understand the interactions of medications, interpersonal relations to communicate effectively, and team building to give our patients the best overall care so everyone is on the same page.

There is a lot to be learned from books and articles; however, I wanted to give you thoughts and opinions of nurses who interact with new-to-practice and transitioning nurses every day.

SUCCESS STORY

Kelly Gallagher, MSN, RN-BC, NE-BC

Director, Nurse Residency Program, Penn Medicine, Philadelphia, Pennsylvania.

Please share your thoughts on mentorship, including benefits of the mentorship experience to both mentee and mentor, how to build a relationship with a mentor, how to be a great mentee.

I believe mentorship is essential for nurses at all levels. Mentees are able to build relationships, advance careers, and receive coaching and professional advice from his or her mentor. For mentors, there is great value in developing another nurse professionally. There are opportunities to teach, share, and provide wisdom gained to newer nurses. Building relationships with a mentor starts with developing mutually agreed-upon goals. The mentoring relationship must be defined with achievable goals within a set time frame. Being a great mentee starts with commitment and honesty and ends with great advice, career development, and a life-long relationship.

Mentors allow nurses to grow, succeed, and remain in nursing. Mentors are rewarded by grooming another nurse. Mentorship provides benefits to more than just the mentor and mentee. Patients benefit indirectly from the mentor–mentee relationship as does the health system or hospital. Mentors can assist the mentees with any patient problems they may have, which improves patient care. The mentor may do this directly or by finding another nurse to assist the mentee with their specific patient care dilemma. Mentors also help the mentee understand and discover the political canvas of the hospital or health system. This may help the mentee advance their career, but it also ensures that the mentee remains within the health system. The return on investment, or ROI, of a mentoring relationship can be great for the mentor, mentee, and the health system (K. Gallagher, personal communication, August 22, 2019).

What is a preceptor?

A preceptor is defined as a teacher, instructor, or tutor (Dictionary.com, n.d.). You can see how the terms mentor and preceptor are easily used interchangeably. When you are new to a unit and assigned a preceptor to help you through orientation, you need to realize a few things about your preceptor. Your preceptor was asked by the nurse manager to share their knowledge and make you comfortable in your transition from student to new RN or from one unit/specialty to another. Your manager has trust and confidence in your preceptor. Your preceptor may have attended several classes to learn the best way to teach and give feedback. They know how important your orientation is to you and to the unit. Preceptors want you to be successful and learn to give the highest quality patient care; after all that is the goal of nursing!

The amount of knowledge and information in nursing today far exceeds what can be taught through traditional educational programs. This is where preceptors and mentors become invaluable. According to Crew (2016), "precepting involves direct supervision of a novice practitioner for a finite period of time; it is a practical teaching tool" (p. 201). A preceptor provides "timely and constructive feedback on clinical and technical professional development" (Crew, 2016, p. 201). Your preceptor is usually the first person you meet when you arrive on your first day of work. He or she will usually start your orientation with a tour of the unit, introduce you to your new colleagues and other staff, and start you on your new journey.

Effective preceptors are confident in their own abilities, knowledge, and skills and are willing to share their successes with new nurses. Preceptors are skilled clinicians and possess a varied knowledge base. A good preceptor should provide structured learning experiences during orientation. Clinical competence is assessed and developed during orientation. One way to structure a learning experience could be through the use of checklists as a guide to fully develop skills for a specific procedure or caring for a specific group of patients. For example, checklists can be used to help the orientee perform a thorough assessment, care for a patient with a chest tube, or navigate the use of barcodes for medication administration. A preceptor ensures that patient care will improve on the unit by building confidence and competence in their orientees.

When you are asked to be a preceptor, I have a few words of advice. As a preceptor you help the orientee navigate the culture and norms of the unit. Staff communication can be a challenge, especially for a nurse who is new to your unit. You should role model your communication with physicians, nurses, the unit secretary, nursing assistants, and others. Being professional is learned through your role modeling. Professionalism involves demonstrating respect for other nurses, staff, and patients. Your communication is what the new nurse will remember. Remember, becoming a good preceptor takes experience. To succeed you need support from your manager and colleagues. I have found that simulation, case studies, and role play are great techniques for a preceptor to use to help the new nurse to think critically in a safe environment. New nurses can get overwhelmed and feel that nursing is not for them. Retention is a concern and consideration for all hospitals. As a preceptor, you should be interested in keeping your orientee as a part of your unit for consistency in patient care.

Not all preceptor–preceptee relationships are a perfect match. I asked Kelly Gallagher how she deals with mismatched preceptors and preceptees.

How do you deal with a novice nurse who is paired with the wrong preceptor? Could you give an anonymous example?

If a nurse resident is struggling with a preceptor, we coach the nurse resident with three simple strategies: speak up, advocate for yourself, and communicate. Early on in the Nurse Residency Program, we teach our nurse residents their preferred "learning style" and advise them to have a discussion with their preceptor. If the match is not working well, we suggest advocating for himself or herself with unit leaders and preceptors and recognizing that there might be a mismatch in learning styles between the preceptor and preceptee. Communicating often with the unit leaders and preceptors is recommended. We suggest novice nurses complete a Daily Rewind, focusing on what went well today, what could have been done differently, what areas need further knowledge/education, and areas of focus for the next shift.

We had a new graduate nurse working on a medical-surgical unit. She shared with the nurse residency team that she is a kinesthetic learner and her preceptor is a read/write learner. She was struggling to communicate with her preceptor and felt as though her orientation was not progressing as it should. She felt as though she should be learning more, practicing more, and felt as though her preceptor was not giving her the independence that she needed. After coaching her to speak up and communicate with her preceptor, our new graduate nurse advocated for herself and was able to develop mutually agreed-upon check-ins with her preceptor. She would share her plan with her preceptor, discuss rationale, and learn using her kinesthetic style. She completed orientation (as scheduled) and now has a great working relationship with her preceptor (K. Gallagher, personal communication, August 22, 2019).

I have been a nurse for quite some time and have had relationships with both preceptors and mentors, beginning with my diploma in nursing, BSN, MSN, and DNP. Every experience was different, and I learned something from each person. I took a position in a new hospital, and my preceptor was younger than me and had less experience in the specialty. She was very nervous and told me that she thought that I would actually teach her. My response was easy: I would share my knowledge about the specialty if she would share her knowledge about the culture of the unit and how to maneuver the charting system. Please remember that you are the specialist of your unit when you become a preceptor.

ADULT LEARNING THEORY

Malcolm Knowles, an American educator, is credited with the use of the term "androgagy" as the art and science of adult learning (Pappas, 2013). Knowles stated that adult learners are self-directed, ready to learn, and motivated (Learning Theory, 2017). Preceptors and mentors alike need to recognize that new and experienced nurses need to be involved in the planning of their education and orientation. New nurses want to know that what they are learning has immediate relevance to their work life. There is a need to explain the reasons specific procedures are being taught. Orientees want to know the reason that the procedure was ordered for this patient. The preceptor should help the new nurse to think critically; instruction should be disease or procedure specific as applied to patient care. The nurse should "think it through" and not just memorize. The new nurse learned about these diseases and procedures in the vacuum of the classroom and probably never had the chance to apply that knowledge to a patient having that disease or needing that procedure. The preceptor is helping the new nurse to connect the dots. Knowles thought that adults learn best with a preceptor until they have the knowledge and experience to be an independent practitioner.

Preceptor Versus Mentor

The main difference between a preceptor and a mentor is that preceptors are teachers/tutors, while mentors are trusted counselors and guides. A mentor is usually a very experienced nurse, while a preceptor could be practicing for as little as 2 years. New-to-practice nurses will come across many experienced nurses who will influence their careers in different ways.

A preceptor prepares the nurse to work independently on the unit. They ensure that the nurse's skills improve and that they experience a variety of patients throughout orientation. A preceptor models and teaches how the nurse can communicate with the rest of the team. The purpose of orientation is to familiarize the nurse to the policies, procedures, and the culture of the unit. Preceptors assist the nurse with skills and answers their questions while evaluating the accomplishments of the nurse. The precepting relationship ends with the completion of orientation.

A mentoring relationship may be a formal or informal process but needs to be purposeful. Mentors encourage and support so the nurse can grow professionally. Mentors do not judge. Mentors do not evaluate; rather they coach and advise. The relationship between the mentor and the nurse is built on trust.

A preceptorship can last the length of the orientation, which at some institutions may be up to 12 weeks. Mentorship does not have a preset expiration date. A mentoring relationship should last as long as both parties find importance in the situation.

As a preceptor, the expectation is to provide evaluation and feedback, establish clear goals during orientation, and share expertise willingly. As a mentor, the expectation is to supply support in any situation, offer advice, and never be judgmental.

Nurse Residency Program

You have passed your NCLEX-RN® and obtained your first professional job. You attend the general orientation with butterflies in your stomach from both fear and excitement. Now you have been enrolled in something called a nurse residency program with every other new-to-practice nurse. Many healthcare organizations are requiring that new nurses attend this program to help ease the transition into practice and decrease turnover. So, what is a nurse residency program? The program is a formalized orientation lasting usually about 1 year. The new nurse works full time on their unit while receiving specialty training and meeting with other new nurses, on a regular basis, to discuss their successes. According to Twibell (2012), the curriculum and clinical experiences in a nurse residency program are evidence based. This program gives the new nurse a chance for socialization with other members of the healthcare team.

In 2010, the Institute of Medicine (IOM) released a report titled *The Future of Nursing: Leading Change, Advancing Health*. The report concluded that nurses should have the benefit of a residency program to begin their careers and throughout transitions (Bleich, 2012). These programs augment nursing education programs and act as a bridge for the transition to practice.

A residency program complements an orientation in these ways, according to (Bleich, 2012):

- Occurs during a career transition
- Fosters reflection through case reviews
- Advances communication skills and helps the nurse navigate the culture of the organization
- Builds confidence by linking critical thinking with critical actions
- Expands leadership through network building

I work in an institution with a nurse residency program. There are goals and expected outcomes from the program that are established on day one and enforced throughout the program. Nurses in the residency program must form small teams, discover a problem on their unit, and solve it through evidence-based methods. These solutions are submitted to the ANCC annual conference to be considered as a podium presentation or as a poster. They also come to the simulation center to practice patient advocacy while learning new skills.

Another question for Kelly Gallagher:

What is ANCC's definition of nurse residency?

The ANCC, one of the two accrediting bodies for nurse residency programs, defines a nurse residency program as "a transition program for nurses with less than 12 months experience." Penn Medicine is accredited by the Commission on Collegiate Nursing Education (CCNE) and defines nurse residency as a series of learning sessions and other experiences that occurs continuously over a 12-month period, and that is designed to assist new participants as they transition to their first professional nursing role. Intended for direct care roles in the healthcare organization, the program is offered by a healthcare organization in partnership with an academic nursing program(s). Only new graduates of prelicensure nursing programs are eligible to participate in the residency program (K. Gallagher, personal communication, August 22, 2019).

What are your retention rates since instituting the program?

Penn Medicine started as one of six hospitals in the United States to partner with University HealthSystem Consortium (UHC)/AACN, now Vizient/AACN, to develop the nurse residency program in 2002. Penn Medicine's total retention rate for 2018 was 92.5%. We are benchmarked against other Vizient/AACN nurse residency programs. The retention rate for nurse residents participating in the Vizient program is 91.5% compared to the national retention rate of 71% (K. Gallagher, personal communication, August 22, 2019).

HOW DO YOU FIND A MENTOR?

Good mentors come in all ages, genders, and races. You want to look for a mentor not by what they do but by the way they do it (Rolfe, 2017, p. 41). There are mentors for any of your needs or phases of your career. You need to consider what type of mentoring you need. So, how do you find a mentor? Two words: network and observation. As you network, someone knows someone who may be right for you, so ask your friends and colleagues. Observation is another way to find your mentor. Who role models the characteristics you think are needed to be successful? Pay attention to people you admire and ask them to be your mentor. Remember that as you ask someone to be your mentor, be open to their answer. Do not be disappointed if now is not a good time to devote to or include you in their life. You do not know what is happening in their personal or professional life. You may be surprised that they will call you when they are free to start a mentoring relationship.

Consider finding someone who can challenge your thinking, someone who listens thoughtfully and who helps to clarify your vision. Remember that a good mentor will be different from you as your differences offer the most for self-development.

Rolfe (2017) lists several types of mentors/mentoring:

1. Traditional mentoring: The mentor has experience in a specific area of nursing or has achieved something you would like to achieve, shares their knowledge, or provides resources to help you advance.
2. Role model: Someone whose behaviors and strategies you can emulate to achieve success in nursing.

3. Developmental mentoring: Someone who listens and challenges you to achieve your goals. They can help you create a plan and make decisions.
4. Reciprocal mentoring: Neither party is labeled as the mentor. Each of you is a resource to the other. You each listen and advise while sharing experiences.
5. Group mentoring: Find collective wisdom and obtain mutual support.
6. Coaching: Personalized training to improve performance. (p. 41)

You do not have to become your mentor. However, people that you know have qualities that you admire or can copy to improve your nursing skills. No one is perfect, and you may want to ignore some less effective aspects of your mentor's behavior. Role models abound; you just need to keep your eyes open. The mentoring process may be considered more important than technical expertise if you are looking for a developmental mentor. You are looking for a mentor who asks you thought-provoking and provocative questions to help clarify your thoughts and vision. A mentor will help you assess alternative strategies or "plan B" as you think of ways to advance your career. If you are looking for some reciprocal mentoring, then you probably have a friend or colleague with whom you share your professional thoughts. Find a peer who may be at the same level as you and experiencing the same things. What you have in common will be beneficial as you both discuss your work environment. Just remember that this is a type of mentoring, not a time for complaining without solutions. In group mentoring, everyone benefits from the shared wisdom. A coach is not necessarily a mentor. Coaches are more specifically used to improve clinical skills and improve performance. However, the relationship can certainly develop into one of mentor–mentee. A good mentor should be different from you as they have unique points of view; otherwise, they would have nothing to offer.

HOW TO BUILD AND NURTURE YOUR RELATIONSHIP WITH A MENTOR

You want your mentor to offer career advice to help you reach your goals. A mentoring relationship takes time to grow; trust takes time to build. Richards (2014) shares a list of five conversation tools to help make a better connection with your mentor each time you meet.

1. Be reliable: Be on time and professional whenever you meet. Your mentor deserves your full attention; it goes a long way to establishing mutual respect.

2. Communicate frequently: It is your responsibility to contact your mentor when you need a sounding board or just need to chat. Listen to your mentor, and take their suggestions to heart. Email or call your mentor when you have updates. I would ask my mentor how often they would like to meet and how frequently they would ike me to email or call. You want to be respectful of your mentor's time.

3. Get personal: Build a rapport. All your conversations do not have to revolve around you and your goals. Remember that your mentor is not your best friend, so keep conversations professional but inclusive of both parties. Getting to know one another goes a long way in building trust. Take your discussion cues from your mentor; they will guide you as to what topics might not be available to discuss.

4. Tap into hindsight: Your mentor has more insight into the profession than you do. Ask your mentor how they got started or how they advanced. Your mentor probably has ideas about which professional organizations you should join and how to get involved, getting the most from the experience. By the way, a professional organization is a great place to meet a prospective mentor. Your goal should be to optimize success in your career.

5. Ask for honesty: Let your mentor know that you are open to feedback. Your mentor needs to know that they can be transparent and honest with you in all aspects of your relationship. (p. 2)

SUCCESS STORY

Jason Gilbert, PhD, MBA, RN, NEA-BC

Executive Vice President and Chief Nurse Executive, Indiana University Health, Indianapolis, Indiana

Jason Gilbert shares his nursing experience and highlights his mentor–mentee moments. Dr. Gilbert is an excellent example of working one's way to the top!

Provide highlights of your professional nursing journey. What are key things that helped you succeed to achieve your professional goals?

I started my career as a staff nurse on an oncology unit. Even as a new nurse, I gravitated toward informal leadership roles. Within the first year I precepted many students and learned the charge nurse role. I participated in unit committees and was usually the first to volunteer to learn a new care protocol or care for a new patient population. I had a great group of mentors in my first role that were interested in my development and a great manager who encouraged and empowered me to get involved.

I loved the work that I did and then met and fell in love with my wife, who is also a nurse. Shortly after getting married, we decided to become travel nurses. We worked in several different states and many different health systems. Although we originally did travel nursing for the fun and variety of living in different places, it was incredibly enriching profession- ally. I experienced a variety of settings, had more exposure to diverse populations, and learned the differences in working for academic, urban, community, for-profit, and not-for profit hospitals. I learned a great deal from experiencing different organizational structures and leadership styles. I learned the areas in which I most liked providing care.

After traveling for several years, we returned to Ohio and worked on a cardiothoracic surgical unit. I was approached by the manager (who became my next great mentor) about considering a career in leadership because of the qualities she saw in my interactions with patients and staff. I took an assistant nurse manager position and grew to love the leadership role. After a year I progressed to a nurse manager position and loved the role. After becoming a manager, I met with the chief nurs- ing officer (CNO), who became a great mentor and encouraged me to get involved in organizational initiatives and encouraged me to go back to school to complete my master's degree. I completed my MBA while working as a manager and found that my leadership abilities were greatly enhanced by the application of what I had learned. While I was complet- ing my MBA, the CNO left the organization for another opportunity but remained a close mentor. After graduation, the same CNO recruited me to a director-level role at a different hospital.

While in the director role, the CNO again encouraged me to return to school. I completed my PhD in 2017. The PhD journey was extremely rich, and I was able to learn to think differently about systems of care and engaging in research and better enculturation of an evidence-based practice (EBP) framework. Shortly after I completed my doctoral work, the CNO left for another opportunity, and I assumed the CNO role at my current organization. This has been a great opportunity for learning, growth, and development in leading a very large team.

I would be remiss if I also didn't give credit to the many people I have worked with along the way and my very strong support system I have from my wife, daughter, and family, who are very supportive of my career goals. These are the people who have most influenced my life, my career, and my success through their love and support.

As a new graduate nurse, did you envision yourself being where you are right now in your career? Include advice for nurses who are just starting in their careers or who find themselves at the crossroads of their career.

Of course I never thought I would be where I am in my career. I think that the more you experience, the more you realize that even the best-laid plans do not always work out as you thought they would, but the lessons you learn in the journey make the journey worth taking. I always joke that I still don't know what I want to be when I grow up. I think part of continued growth and development is self-reflecting on your relevance in your team and organization and being open to possibilities.

As far as advice for nurses who are starting their career or those at a crossroads, I can say one of the most valuable lessons I have learned is the following: It is not about you. It is really about the team and the patients that you serve. The minute you take yourself too seriously is the moment you will make a big mistake. The path to "success" in your career is rarely (if ever) linear. There will be setbacks, failures, and a million miles of roads that you don't currently see. Embrace those and learn from them. When you fail, and you most certainly will at something, ask yourself, "What have I learned from this?" and then move forward. Don't let the fear of failure stop you from trying. Be open to new opportunities, and never let the opportunity to learn something new to pass you by. Never stop learning new things, and continue to learn from those you care for and those your work with. Engage with a mentor you can trust. Admit your mistakes and say you are sorry when necessary. It is acceptable to not always have the answers. The team you are on wants to help you. Remember to take time for yourself and your family.

Please share your thoughts on mentorship, including benefits to both mentee and mentor, how to build a relationship with a metor, and how to be a great mentee.

Engaging with a mentor is one of the single-most important things you can do for yourself to help with your professional development. Do not be afraid to ask someone to be your mentor. I have always found that most people are interested in helping others grow and develop. I have had great mentors from a variety of industries throughout my career and scholarly work, both formal and informal. I have also had the opportunity to mentor many others at various phases of their career.

The cornerstone of the mentor–mentee relationship is trust, honesty, and confidentiality. The relationship needs to be a safe space for both the mentor and mentee to be open and honest with each other. The relationship is reciprocal, and both the mentor and the mentee must be active participants in the relationship for it to be most effective. The mentor must give honest feedback and guidance, keep sensitive topics or struggles in confidence, help the mentee with self-reflection and discovery, act in the best interest of the mentee, and provide advice and suggestions without telling or solving every problem for the mentee. The mentor provides a safe space for the mentee to be their authentic self and to explore difficult topics. They also serve in part as a champion and protector of the mentee and take an active part in their growth and development. The mentee in turn is not a passive participant in the process. They also must be honest, be open to giving and receiving feedback, and hold in confidence difficult issues that are discussed. The mentee has just as much ownership for the relationship and needs to manage the relationship actively to ensure that it is effective. While many mentor programs are formal, the relationship cannot always be "forced," and the mentor and mentee should both ensure that they are a match. As with any relationship, there is a beginning where the relationship is forming and patterns of interactions are established, a middle where the relationship is in full effect, and an ending where the relationship transitions. Often the mentor and mentee relationship transitions to a professional friendship after the relationship transitions to the next phase.

The mentors I have had throughout my career have greatly contributed to my success. I have had many different mentors throughout my career in different industries. Each of these people has had the qualities that I have mentioned. They have challenged me, guided me, and helped me to see things in myself that I didn't necessarily see. They have helped me through struggles and have helped to celebrate in my successes. Many of the relationships have transitioned to great friendships as I have progressed in my career, and I have stayed connected to most of the mentors I have had the opportunity to engage with.

Although there is much focus on the value that the mentee receives, as a mentor I know that I have received just as much value in mentoring others. It is a great responsibility to help others in their development, and I always learn about different perspectives. And I always learn just as much (if not more) from my mentees as they learn from me. I believe that mentoring others keeps you current, challenges your thinking, and helps you to learn about others. Often, I receive great advice from mentees about my leadership or important decisions that need to be made (J. Gilbert, personal communication, July 25, 2019).

SUCCESS STORY

Cara Davis, MSN, RN, CCRN

Clinical Practice Lead IV, MICU, Hospital of the University of Pennsylvania, Philadelphia

Cara Davis is a Clinical Nurse III in a large academic medical center's medical intensive care unit (MICU). Note that this MICU has preceptors plus a program for nurses to find a mentor. Cara said that during the onboarding phases of new-to-practice nurses, preceptors are chosen based on willingness to precept, completion of a system-wide class to develop preceptors, and a personality similarity between the new nurse and the staff nurse. The preceptor is responsible for ensuring the new nurse is meeting the benchmarks of providing safe and effective patient care. There are weekly objectives, guidelines, and policies that course this instruction and evaluation. The MICU has a current voluntary mentorship program that is available to all new staff. If they would like to seek out mentorship in addition to their primary preceptor, there is a shared drive that has biographies of all willing staff to provide mentorship. The new hire can view each biography and select the mentor based on what the new nurse would consider to be meaningful to them. Whether it is geographic location, personal goals, or hobbies, there have been several new staff members who have sought mentorship through this channel, and both individuals have phone conversations, coffee and/or lunch breaks together. There is a nurse who comes to mind that had sought out a mentor aside from her preceptor. This nurse was struggling to feel like she was "fitting in." She was meeting the objectives of her orientation and was providing safe patient care but just was unsure if she was the right fit for the unit. Her mentor and she would meet weekly, usually off the unit, in their spare time. The mentor later shared with me, with the approval of the mentee, that their meetings aided in her overall success in the unit. The mentor was able to share similar experiences of how she felt as a new nurse coming to the MICU. She was able to validate many of the new nurse's feelings, making her feel as though this was all part of a normal transition process. The new nurse is thriving on the unit today. She has been on the unit for a couple of years and is requesting to be a preceptor so that she can also help guide and mentor a new nurse starting on the unit (C. Davis, personal communication, August 21, 2019).

Personal Reflection on My Mentorship Experience

I have been fortunate to have several wonderful mentors throughout my career. When I left my staff position on a medical-surgical unit and started working in a medical intensive care unit (MICU), Mary, my preceptor, became my mentor. Mary was intelligent and kind and calm during every situation. I was confident in my knowledge and care on my previous unit, but everything in the ICU seemed larger than life. I found myself feeling unsure and more than just a little apprehensive in the beginning. I do not usually use either of those adjectives to describe myself. Mary taught me how to be a "unit nurse" but always credited me for my previous knowledge. She started asking me about my future plans. Mary received her MSN when most nurses in that hospital only achieved their BSN. When we had a break during my orientation, she would tell me about all of the possible next steps she could see me taking to help move the profession forward. I stayed connected to critical care throughout my career and remembered Mary's words as I achieved my MSN and became a clinical nurse specialist, accepted a faculty position, and received my DNP. I may not have thought of changing my professional trajectory had Mary not planted the seed.

Final Note on Mentorship

Cara Davis gives an example of mentorship through professional development:

There is a nurse on our unit who had a great idea geared toward providing mentorship through developing a day enriched with 1:1 support as well as skill development. Initial phases of this idea lacked support from our leadership team on the unit at that time. With a change in leadership and creation of a new role, clinical practice lead (CPL), there was partnership with this nurse to get this idea developed and implemented. With the mentorship of the CPL and the bedside nurse, the mentorship day was developed into something much larger and meaningful than initial phases. Together we were able to hold the day off campus, in the Simulation Center, and offer guest speakers, hands-on training, as well as 1:1 dialogue and case studies. We reached out to our educational department and offered CEUs for the day as well. Due to the mentorship, this bedside nurse has advanced her clinical ladder using this as a launching pad. She is also currently nominated for Distinguished Nurse Clinician based on her eagerness and willingness to ensure safe patient care through the development of new staff (C. Davis, personal communication, August 21, 2019).

CONCLUSION

Mentoring, done the right way, results in competent and confident nurses achieving their professional goals. A successful mentorship requires commitment and is anchored in trust and openness. The mentor and mentee set clear goals, timelines, and milestones. Both pledge to fulfill the plan and engage in a supportive and reciprocal relationship.

Key Points

- A mentor is someone who can help guide you through your professional journey.
- A mentor shares their knowledge, so pay it forward and become a mentor yourself.
- No matter where you are in your career—beginning, middle, or near the end—a mentor will always be helpful.

References

Bleich, M. (2012). In praise of nursing residency programs. *American Nurse Today, 7*(5). Retrieved from https://www.americannursetoday.com/in-praise-of-nursing-residency-programs/

Crew, R. (2016). Personality and mentoring: Stepping off on the right foot. *The Journal of Continuing Education in Nursing, 47*(5), 201–203. doi:10.3928/00220124-20160419-02

Dictionary.com. (n.d.). *Mentor*. Retrieved from https://www.dictionary.com/browse/mentor?s=t

Everwise. (2015). *From Oprah to Churchill: 20 inspiring mentoring quotes.* Retrieved from https://www.geteverwise.com/mentoring/20-inspiring-mentorship-quotes/

Hnatiuk, C. (2013). Mentoring nurses toward success. *Minority Nurse*. Retrieved from https://minoritynurse.com/mentoring-nurses-toward-success/

Learning Theories. (2017). Andragogy—Adult learning theory (Knowles). *Learning Theories*. Retrieved from https://www.learning-theories.com/andragogy-adult-learning-theory-knowles.html

Merriam-Webster.com. (n.d.). *Mentor.* Retrieved from https://www.merriam-webster.com/dictionary/mentor

Montavio, W., & Veenema, T. (2015). Mentorship in developing transformational leaders to advance health policy: Creating a culture of health. *Nurse Leader, 13*(1), 65–69. doi:10.1016/j.mnl.2014.05.020

Pappas, C. (2013). *The adult learning theory—Andragogy—of Malcolm Knowles.* https://elearningindustry.com/the-adult-learning-theory-andragogy-of-malcolm-knowles

Richards, K. (2014). *5 conversation tools for nurturing your relationship with a mentor.* Retrieved from https://www.forbes.com/sites/85broads/2014/07/29/5-conversation-tools-for-nurturing-your-relationship-with-a-mentor/#2af796ef510d

Rolfe, A. (2017). What to look for in a mentor. *Korean Journal of Medical Education, 29,* 41–43. doi:10.3946/KJME.2017.52

Shaikh, A. M. (2017). Understanding effective mentoring in nursing education: The relational-reliant concept. *JOJ Nurse Health Care, 2*(5), 555596. Retrieved from https://juniperpublishers.com/jojnhc/pdf/JOJNHC.MS.ID.555596.pdf

Stanford Health Care Mentoring Program. (2019). *Nursing: Professional development.* Retrieved from https://stanfordhealthcare.org/health-care-professionals/nursing/professional-development/mentorship.html

Twibell, R. (2012). *Tripping over the welcome mat: Why new nurses don't stay and what the evidence says we can do about it.* Retrieved from https://www.americannursetoday.com/tripping-over-the-welcome-mat-why-new-nurses-dont-stay-and-what-the-evidence-says-we-can-do-about-it/

7

Becoming an Expert

Rhoda R. Redulla

"I am most proud of my ability to connect with people in very vulnerable states. To be entrusted with informing people of risks, benefits, known medical treatments and most effective treatments. To open my gift of knowledge to teach families and communities be fully aware partners in their own care."

—Suzanne Rubin, DNP, MPH, CRNP-P

It's never too late to be who you want to be. You may find yourself at the crossroads of your career, questioning if it is worth pursuing a higher degree or a major career goal. Should you do it or wait?

It is a major decision to pursue further education, involving time, money, and a staunch commitment to complete the required work. Becoming an expert requires time and positive persistence. This chapter provides additional insight about what it takes to pursue further education in nursing or to accomplish a new credential such as being certified in a nursing specialty.

WHY PURSUE FURTHER EDUCATION: THE GLOBAL VIEW

One of the key messages in the 2010 Institute of Medicine (IOM) *The Future of Nursing: Leading Change, Advancing Health* report was that nurses should achieve higher levels of education and training through an improved education system that promotes seamless academic progression. Care, regardless of setting, is increasingly becoming more complex with sicker patients, having multiple comorbidities, including chronic illnesses. Innovation and swift development of new technology to deliver patient care will keep being a mainstay in healthcare. To continue to provide appropriate care, the IOM recommended that nurses with baccalaureate or BSN degrees should increase to 80% in 2020. An increase in the proportion of nurses with a BSN also would create a workforce poised to achieve higher levels of education at the master's and doctoral levels, required for nurses to serve as primary care providers, nurse researchers, and nurse faculty. Having a baccalaureate degree would also allow nurses to pursue and make an impact in other areas such as health policy and healthcare financing, community and public health, leadership, quality improvement, and systems thinking (IOM, 2011). To support this goal, RN-to-BSN programs were created. The RN-to-BSN program is intended for RNs who completed a diploma or associate in nursing program. Many organizations have modified their existing tuition benefit program in response to the IOM report. Some government agencies established grants by forging academic and practice partnerships for nurse practitioner (NP) programs. The Health Resources and Services Administration (HRSA), a federal agency within the U.S. Department of Health and Human Services, is tasked for improving healthcare to people who are geographically isolated and economically or medically vulnerable. It provides funding for several programs that support the education and practice of advanced practice registered nurses (APRNs). Advanced Nursing Education Workforce (ANEW) is just one of the several programs that HRSA supports. The ANEW program supports academic clinical partnerships to educate and graduate primary care NPs, clinical nurse specialists (CNSs), and nurse midwives (NMs) who are academically and clinically prepared for the unique challenges of transitioning from nursing school to practice in rural and underserved communities (HRSA, 2019).

In 2019, the American Association of Colleges of Nursing (AACN) released a position statement that calls for supporting pathways that will support RNs with associate degrees and diplomas into programs leading to a baccalaureate degree (or entry-level master's degree) offered by an accredited 4-year college or university (AACN, 2019). The AACN stated that supporting academic progression at the baccalaureate level is also key to meeting the nation's demand for APRNs, nursing school faculty, nurse researchers, and leaders.

In response to the growing interest in developing an alternative to the research-focused doctorates, PhD in nursing or DNSc (Doctor of Nursing Science), the AACN created a task force to develop standards for a new DNP program in 2004. The 11-member task force reviewed the literature and obtained input from key groups (deans, program directors, students) at the eight current or planned practice-focused doctoral programs at the time. The task force developed recommendations and identified essential elements of the curriculum for the DNP program.

Since the inception of the program, employers are quickly recognizing the value and unique contribution of DNP-prepared nurses in the practice arena (AACN, 2019). DNP-prepared nurses lead initiatives that improve patient, population, and organizational outcomes. They lead strategic initiatives to influence policy. There is a growing demand for DNP-prepared nurses. As of 2019, 348 DNP programs are currently enrolling students at schools of nursing nationwide, and an additional 98 new DNP programs are in the planning stages (50 postbaccalaureate and 48 postmaster's programs).

WHY PURSUE FURTHER EDUCATION: THE ORGANIZATIONAL VIEW

Although there is limited evidence on the impact of postgraduate study and improved patient outcomes, a better educated workforce has clear advantages. Current evidence suggests that nurses who pursue postgraduate study are more likely to have improved critical thinking and decision-making skills, demonstrate leadership qualities to empower them to challenge poor practice, and have the skills needed for advanced clinical practice roles. The *Future of Nursing* report (IOM, 2011) discusses the need to ensure that nurses are educated to assume leadership roles across the system in order to tackle the challenges ahead in redesigning the facets of healthcare delivery. Nurses with a DNP make vital contributions in healthcare. They help assess critical situations that arise in clinical practice and develop programs and solutions to address them.

Suzanne Rubin, a DNP-prepared neonatal nurse practitioner featured later in this chapter, demonstrated how she grew and developed in her DNP program. The DNP program has an intensive and research-based framework, that culminates in a scientific project that draws from existing medical literature and observation. The DNP project allows nurses to create structure to an organic way of thinking that comes naturally for critically thinking nurses (McComas, 2011).

In Suzanne's words, "I knew how to think that way, but I didn't know how to use evidence to make a point and influence care." Her DNP project aimed to reduce the negative outcomes for which late preterm infants (34–36 weeks of gestation) are at risk, including hyperbilirubinemia, prolonged hospital length of stay, feeding difficulties, and associated weight loss. Suzanne developed a late-preterm specialized order set consisting of five specific, research-proven interventions. After implementation, her project was later reviewed by the Perinatal Cooperative and Maryland's Department of Health and Hygiene.

WHY PURSUE FURTHER EDUCATION: THE PERSONAL VIEW

Whether it is going back to school for an RN-to-BSN program or a master's degree or a doctoral degree, there are clear benefits of education. An article posted on nursejournal.org (2020) cited 25 reasons for why to pursue a master's degree in nursing. I have selected a few of them and provided more insight in this section.

Obtain Greater Knowledge

Going back to school provides an opportunity to broaden your knowledge on topics that you have not learned in your basic nursing education. In a master's program, you can pursue advanced clinical knowledge and skills through a NP or nurse anesthesia program. Suzanne Rubin, DNP, featured in a success story later in this chapter, was inspired by her work with vulnerable children and moved on to pursue a master's degree, neonatal nurse practitioner program. At the time she pursued her master's degree, Suzanne was working in a pediatric clinical research unit. She was involved in conducting research on pediatric allergy, genetics, HIV, and infectious diseases, alongside some of the most brilliant physician scientists. This experience spurred Suzanne's drive to learn more and do more.

Pursue a New Specialty

Many nurses go back to school to pursue a new specialty. Clinical trials, nursing education, leadership—these are just some options for you to pursue. Another colleague recently completed a master's degree in holistic nursing. She was working in a rehabilitation unit and saw how patients could grow dependent on pharmacologic measures to alleviate their pain and anxiety. This spurred her interest in holistic methods of intervention and she decided to take her interest a step further by applying for a master's program.

Expand Your Network

When you go back to school, you meet new people and expand your professional network. During my doctoral program, exceptional opportunities opened up to me, including being invited to coauthor a book chapter. One of my professors was involved in a publication project and happened to be looking for an author along my line of specialty. This experience introduced me to the world of book publishing and prompted me to stay connected with my professional organization.

Higher Earning Potential

With a higher degree, you increase your chances of having higher pay. Although salary can be a low motivator for professional development

(Horn, Pilkington, & Hooten, 2019), a nurse's earning potential increases with a higher degree (Hagan & Curtis, 2018).

More Respect in the Field and From Peers

With an advanced or specialized education, you become known as an expert in your field. A former colleague who pursued her DNP degree took up her interest in the implementation of a nursing peer feedback process. She reviewed the best and current evidence on the best practices in peer feedback, conducted an assessment of her own organization where she had planned to carry out her capstone project, and developed a plan. Her intervention included an educational program on how to provide and receive feedback from peers and proceeded to implement the complete peer feedback process on selected units at the hospital. After completing her degree, she disseminated her work within and outside the organization by presenting in conferences.

More Career Options

When Brian, a critical care nurse, decided to go for an MSN degree, his unit recently did a pilot run of a new acuity tool specific for the nonverbal patient. Brian was fascinated with how nurses from the informatics team translated the tool into a convenient electronic tool. His interest in a nursing informatics career was sparked by the innovative work of his hospital's informatics department. Brian had the opportunity to explore nursing career options with the nurses on the informatics team, and shortly thereafter, he started looking into MSN nursing informatics programs. Completing further education presents more options to engage in other work fields within nursing.

NURSING ACADEMIC PROGRAMS

RN-to-BSN

The RN-to-BSN degree program is designed for nurses who have their RN licensure and aim to obtain a BSN degree. The BSN degree prepares nurses for a broader scope of practice and helps them to develop their clinical, leadership, and scientific inquiry skills (Lesh, 2016).

BSN in 10 Bill

In December 2017, New York State was the first to pass a "BSN in 10" bill requiring nurses to have a baccalaureate degree. According to the bill, "in order to continue to maintain registration as a registered professional nurse in New York state, [nurses must] have attained a

BOX 7.1 RN-TO-BSN SAMPLE CURRICULUM

Prerequisites
English Composition (3 credits)
General Psychology (3 credits)
General Chemistry (3 credits) and Laboratory (3 credits)
Microbiology (3 credits) and Laboratory (1 credit)
Human Anatomy and Physiology 1 and 2 (6 credits)
and Laboratory
Introduction to Sociology (3 credits)
Statistics (3 credits)

Completion Curriculum
Professional Nursing Science (3 credits)
Health Assessment (3 credits)
Aging and Health (3 credits)
Information Technology: Applications in Health Care (2 credits)
Transformational Leadership (3 credits)
Research Basis of Nursing (3 credits)
Nursing Electives

baccalaureate degree or higher in nursing within 10 years of initial licensure" (New York State Senate, 2017).

Section 3 of the bill takes effect 18 months after the act became law. Current RNs, nursing students, or those pending acceptance into a program preparing RNs on the effective date of this act (which was December 19, 2017) were grandfathered in. This means they are exempt from the provisions of the bill. Current RNs who are grandfathered in are encouraged to take their BSN. Nurses who plan to complete their BSN can inquire about tuition reimbursement programs in their facility and flexible work hours. Some schools also offer online programs and may be the best option for nurses who have child care needs.

The bill is in conjunction with the IOM recommendation for nurses to achieve a higher level of education. Patients' needs have become more complex. To respond to these changes, requisite competencies are needed, including leadership, health policy, system improvement, research and evidence-based practice, and teamwork and collaboration.

Master's Degree in Nursing

Several pathways are available for nurses desiring to pursue a master's degree. MSN degrees are offered to eligible nurses with interest in either clinical, leadership, or informatics education (Box 7.2).

BOX 7.2 MSN DEGREE OPTIONS

Advanced Role Tracks

- Clinical Nurse Leader
- Research/Clinical Trials
- Leadership and Healthcare Administration
- Nursing Education
- Clinical Nurse Specialist

Nurse Practitioner

- Adult Gerontology Acute Care Nurse Practitioner
- Adult Gerontology Primary Care Nurse Practitioner
- Family Nurse Practitioner (Individual Across the Lifespan)
- Pediatric Acute Care Nurse Practitioner
- Pediatric Primary Care Nurse Practitioner
- Pediatric Primary/Pediatric Acute Nurse Practitioner Dual Program
- Psychiatric-Mental Health Nurse Practitioner
- Women's Health/Gender-Related Nurse Practitioner
- Nurse Anesthesia
- Nurse Midwife

Nurses may also opt to go for nonnursing degrees, such an MBA, MPH, or MBE, and acquire knowledge and skills in these specific areas.

Post-Master's Certificate

A post-master's certificate option is also available to nurses already having a master's degree and wishing to pursue another area of specialty. A current NP colleague who was encouraged to be a clinical preceptor wanted to advance her skills in instruction. She pursued a post-master's certificate in nursing education. Today, she is still a practicing NP and employed as an adjunct faculty on a part-time basis. She claims she found her "dream job": teaching while continuing to practice. The post-master's certification option is offered in many other specialties, such as nursing informatics and advanced practice nurse roles.

Doctoral Degree in Nursing

Two doctoral nursing degree options are available: PhD and DNP. Are you looking to enroll in a doctoral program and find yourself

Table 7.1

	DNP/PhD/DNS Contrast Grid	
	DNP	**PhD/DNS**
Program of Study	Objectives: Prepare nurse leaders at the highest level of nursing practice to improve patient outcomes and translate research into nursing practice	Objectives: Prepare nurses at the highest level of nursing science to conduct research to advance the science of nursing
Students	■ Commitment to practice career ■ Oriented toward improving outcomes of patient care and population health	■ Commitment to research career ■ Oriented toward developing new nursing knowledge and scientific inquiry

Source: Reproduced with permission from the American Association of Colleges of Nursing. (n.d.). *DNP education.* Retrieved from https://www.aacnnursing.org/Nursing-Education-Programs/DNP-Education

perplexed in choosing the right terminal degree? If you are more inclined toward research, then pursue a PhD. If your interest is focused more in advancing practice, then go for your DNP. The following grid from the AACN illustrates key areas of difference in DNP and PhD preparation (Table 7.1).

BARRIERS IN PURSUING AN ADVANCED DEGREE

Financial Requirement

The primary barriers to professional development identified by many nurses are family commitments and financial requirements (Horn et al., 2019). If you decide to pursue further education, speak with your family and lay out the plan on what type of support you will need. For financial requirements, inquire on incentives you can access at work.

Time Constraints

Schools revealed that for every one credit hour in which you enroll, you will spend approximately **2 to 3 hours** per week outside of class studying. Therefore, to help determine the course load most appropriate for you, use this formula: **3 credit hours** (1 course) = **3 hours** in class per week = **6 to 9 hours** study time per week (https://www

.umflint.edu/advising/surviving_college). Take this into consideration and factor your personal circumstances into this requirement. Reach out to another colleague and ask for pointers. When I was pursuing my graduate degree, I had to skip many social functions. I also had to modify my daughter's bedtime so I can work on school assignments earlier in the evenings.

Lack of Organizational or Leadership Support

We hear some organizations provide support to nurses in pursuing a degree, whether baccalaureate, master's, or doctoral. This comes in the form of either tuition support or flexible scheduling. However, not all do.

Individual or Family Circumstances

As stated earlier, individual or family circumstances can present as a barrier to going back to school. These circumstances may include challenges such as caring for a sick family member or your own children going to college.

SUCCESS STORY

Suzanne Rubin, DNP, MPH, CRNP-P

Nursery Pediatric Nurse Practitioner, Johns Hopkins Hospital, Baltimore

Why nursing?

My professional journey probably began as a curious preteen. I loved looking at anatomy books as well as illustrated science magazines. The association of anatomy as well as health and wellness was a constant fascination to me. I enjoyed human development as well, with a younger sister arriving when I was eight. I loved watching her develop and teaching her new things. I started my first job at a hospital, where there was a program for 11th graders to train as nursing assistants. In the hospital setting, I learned many institutional routines but mostly learned about human suffering. I had never been exposed to this side of humanity. I felt compassion deeply for all the people who were hospitalized and particularly vulnerable. I was offered a part-time job as a nursing assistant when I graduated; I also started nursing school at the same time. I rotated to every unit and landed in pediatrics. So many things have changed since 1978, but still every patient was special. I enjoyed all my colleagues (who seemed to have special traits I could emulate). I started with an associate's degree in Michigan, at Northwestern Michigan College (NMC), and also worked at Munson Medical Center. My biggest influence was Mr. Ken Rose, at NMC, my anatomy and physiology instructor. He taught nurses, pre-med, pre-dent students. I excelled and loved the course-work. After graduation, I worked as an inpatient nurse in a pediatric unit, neonatal unit, and obstetric unit, medical unit, cardiac, and ICU. I became a mom and felt a kinship with young families requiring hospitalization.

Pursuing a BSN

I started a BSN program at 25, at the University of Michigan in Ann Arbor, Michigan. Upon graduation, I felt even more capable to be a nurse. I worked in an infant unit, with dialysis, organ transplant, oncology, and infectious diseases. The people that I met in the University of Michigan program have become lifelong friends, guiding and supporting me through seemingly overwhelming odds of completing the program while working. With every advanced degree, it seemed as if I gained increasing associations with other professionals who I would never have met unless I was in school. As I continued to work throughout every degree, I inspired so many to return to school. My "glow" at the process was communicable.

Pursuing an advanced degree

My motivation for returning to school for an MSN degree was initially tentative. I felt my BSN degree would allow me to influence nursing in a way that involved additional themes of thinking. There I learned theories that inspired me, causing me to deeply understand my influence on health and the inner gift I gave. [I realized] ways I mattered and ways I could change assessments, diagnoses, treatments, evaluations, education, and public health idioms for more than just one patient. I could teach with more confidence. I could brighten understanding in ways that people could conceptualize. I could evaluate new ideas to alter health before it became illness. I wanted to support the community to contribute to health.

Becoming an expert

I was hired as a school nurse for a 10,000-pupil district in Traverse City, Michigan. I worked with many teachers, but also two other nurses, both of whom mentored me in true public health. I felt exuberant on a daily basis. I was consulted frequently by many of my assigned 10 schools but was becoming deeply inspired to offer additional health other than recommending a pediatrician for a child. Health is required to learn. Learning is required to succeed. So many children experienced trauma daily, from lack of parental care to abject abuse or neglect. The children who succeeded had a global cushion that spelled H-E-A-L-T-H. I started chronic health groups for asthma and attention deficit hyperactivity disorder (ADHD). I became an expert witness in the school setting for students with ADHD. I supported families, secretaries, and teachers.

Journey to becoming a neonatal nurse practitioner

My colleagues were shocked when I wanted to become a pediatric nurse practitioner. Over a hundred people had applied for my job. It was highly coveted. I was still "hungry." I was still curious. I was still excited to learn more. At this time in my life, I was struggling through a troubling divorce. Even fearing the trauma my own children suffered, I felt I could offer them an example. I found the process of education stimulating, rewarding, challenging. I was always amazed at the inner growth I could palpate throughout the process (not to mention the exhaustion, difficult assignments, cost, etc.). Often, I thought, "Why can't you just leave this academic chase?" as I entered a new program. I became a certified pediatric nurse practitioner at the age of 36 and at the time worked in a Pediatric Clinical Research Unit. Research offered hope to those children who really needed it. I was involved in amazing protocols and researchers, including Dr. Hugh Sampson (pediatric allergy), Dr. Ada Hamosh (pediatric genetics), and Dr. Rod Willoughby (HIV and infectious diseases). My nursing colleagues were some of the most brilliant and fun ladies I have ever known (Kim Mudd and Sally Noone). Never have I learned so much. My favorite patients included the rescue protocols for oncology: five boys who had Ewing's sarcoma. Oncology gets more successful every day as a result of each study subject's contribution.

Since I was now a pediatric nurse practitioner, and working later as an HIV study coordinator (with Dr. Andrea Ruff and Dr. Jean Anderson), I was involved in research protocols with children with congenitally acquired HIV. I especially enjoyed the pregnant mothers who volunteered for the national studies involving antiretrovirals during pregnancy. They may not know how much they have changed the world by proving the safety of a medicine cocktail that changes risk from 1 out of 4 infants becoming infected to fewer than 1 out of 100. These families were like my own. I attended their deliveries and welcomed their babies to the world.

Second master's degree and DNP degree

My experience with these infants exposed me to the joy of the full-term nursery. While the babies at Johns Hopkins are over 34 weeks, they are often high risk. HIV exposure, prematurity, congenital anomalies, and infections are routine diagnoses. I had somehow completed a master's degree in public health (MPH) prior to this time. What I coveted about this degree were the research designs, use of mathematical calculations to determine effects, and the international exposure. We had group "chats" with our partners in other countries. We all had projects that were completed as a presentation or publication. My mentor was Dr. Frank Witter, who patiently met me weekly throughout my investigation of newborn SGA (small for gestational age) sonographic measurement in fetuses and predictability of SGA size in newborns (postnatal correlation). I loved the data manipulation and predictability. I did not feel the academic advisorship was as excellent as I had hoped. I loved my nursery job. I wanted to contribute scientifically to the field. I wanted to find a way to keep the preterm infants on our unit (and not be transferred to the NICU, where they would be physically separated from their mothers). I met an incredible woman, Mary Terhaar. She had an open meeting about the initiation of a DNP soon being initiated at Johns Hopkins School of Nursing. I waited a year. By then I was ready. I revisited my statistics. I enjoyed the "stretch" of the mind—pairing the test with the question, looking at evidence to consider interventions, providing informed consent, discussing and including my colleagues (although most were not particularly interested—almost threatened). I challenged myself. I challenged my professors. I challenged my colleagues. I had statistically significant results. The topic I chose became incredibly popular; all journals had recently published similar studies and declined my manuscript. I was fine.

The actual processes and journey were my greatest benefit. I have had many difficulties in my life (including breast cancer, divorce, and children of trauma). The best part of pursuing advanced degrees was the ability to find an arena with a group of resilient people who strive to learn as well as make a difference. Most resilient people have encountered duress and have thrived. They all sat beside me. They all showed me we had more commonalities than we had differences. They all inspired me with their enthusiasm, diminishing the struggle.

I felt so invincible with the support of professors who were passionate teachers. When I meet them, I know it immediately. We are kindred souls. Mary Terhaar was the most inspirational program director. Her enthusiasm and curiosity pulled me in. I now forget the long nights of producing papers, manuscripts, analyzing data, and losing network connections. I don't mean to minimize the challenge that an advanced degree brings. It is just that the process and outcome far diminishes the challenge. I have never suppressed the glow that learning has delivered to me.

As a nurse starting out, I would offer myself a little advice. As a nurse, there are so many different ways and places to work that you are always able to find a good fit. You can chisel your way to your perfect job (where you shine and feel appreciated). Advanced degrees are difficult but will always propel you to become a better nurse and person. Flexibility in your position is always available in such areas as public health, teaching, research, and so forth. If you don't like one arena, try another. The job market is usually good, and most facilities offer tuition reimbursement. You may find an easier job anywhere else, but you may never make as much of a difference as a nurse. Looking back, I feel I have touched so many lives in such profound ways. I have discovered some strengths in myself I never dreamed I had. I have been able to view my problems as so small compared to those of many others. I have met so many mentors and "sisters." I am challenged every day. I feel grateful for a good cognitive format to make wise and effective treatment plans.

I am most proud of my ability to connect with people in very vulnerable states. To be entrusted with informing people of risks, benefits, known medical treatments, and most effective treatments. To open my gift of knowledge to teach families and communities be fully aware partners in their own care. To encourage families to expect the type of medical care that is sound, safe, and healing.

DIFFERENT MODALITIES

Now that you have seen the "why," here is a road map on how to do it. What are your options? What are the different modalities available to you? A comparison table of hybrid/blended, online, and face-to-face education is shown in Table 7.2 (Todd et al., 2017). Flexible options are available to you when deciding to enter either a baccalaureate program or graduate degree program. You can select to be in an in-person, online, or hybrid program. For graduate students, some programs are offered in executive style format, intended primarily for the working professional.

Table 7.2

	Comparison of Hybrid, Online, and Face-to-Face Education		
	Hybrid/Blended Instruction	**Online**	**Face-to-Face**
Method of Delivery	Required in-person attendance on specific dates with online work	Solely via a computer program or Internet site	Delivered in person by instructor to students
Benefits	Provides a variety of learning experiences and wider range of content	Student may access course materials at a convenient time and place; online quizzes and activities offer immediate feedback; offers flexibility in scheduling	Allows for group interaction, in-depth discussion with other students, and in-person communication between instructor and student
Disadvantage	Lack of regular in-person interaction with instructor and other students	Lack of opportunity for interactive activities and in-person communication with instructor and other students	Lack flexibility in scheduling; hugely driven by instructor's teaching style

Where Do You Start?

- Attend an information session. This is the best first step I can share with you. At the information session, the school typically presents an overview of the institution and the educational programs offered. If multiple programs are being presented at that time, breakout sessions are also offered to have a better opportunity to learn more about your program of interest. This is also your opportunity to meet future faculty, the admission office staff, and current students.
- Once you have decided which program to take, get key information on the application requirements. Here are typical requirements for applying to an advanced degree.

Admission Requirements for MSN

- Proof of current RN licensure
- Bachelor's degree in nursing from a nationally accredited program with a specified minimum GPA (grade point average)
- Official transcripts of the bachelor's degree in nursing
- Personal statement
- Two letters of reference from professional sources (typically requires that one was from a former professor or supervisor)
- Résumé
- Completed application form and fee

Some schools may or may not require an interview with faculty, GRE testing, or an example of previously written scholarly paper.

It is easy to feel overwhelmed and discouraged. Just focus on the current step you are working on. Stay in conversation with nurses who have successfully completed the program.

Barriers for Nurses to Pursue an Advanced Degree

"When investing in a master's degree, the commitment is deserving of serious consideration, research, and financial planning. Should you go for it? According to area experts, the decision depends upon your career goals and financial health" (Prafder, 2017). Unless you have further study, your growth and movement will be limited.

VALUE OF A NATIONAL SPECIALTY CERTIFICATION

Certification is the formal process by which a certifying body validates a nurse's knowledge, skills, and abilities in a specific role and clinical area of practice (Competency and Credentialing Institute,

2017). It is a formal recognition of a nurse's expertise in a specialty and is associated with improved outcomes (Haskins, Hniatuk, & Yoder, 2011). It can also have personal, professional, and economic benefits for you (Fights, 2015). Here are some perceived benefits of specialty certification by nurses (Leonardi, 2011):

- Enhanced professional credibility
- Evidence of professional commitment
- Feelings of personal accomplishment and satisfaction

In a 2006 and 2008 survey conducted by the Orthopaedic Nurses Certification Board (ONCB), respondents indicated that certification allowed them to (Roberts, 2017):

- Experience personal growth
- Feel more competent in their skills as a professional nurse
- Feel more satisfied as a professional nurse
- Feel more confident in their practice
- Be seen as a credible provider
- Serve as a resource to staff for patient care concerns

How to Become Certified

The journey to nursing specialty certification requires commitment and preparation. Certification programs have specific eligibility requirements in terms of education, experience, and, sometimes, continuing education (Table 7.3).

Advanced practice roles such as NP, nurse anesthetist, CNS, and certified nurse midwife also require specialty certification. For more detailed information, visit the certifying body's website.

How to Prepare for the Certification Test

Planning for Your Study Preparation

- Be familiar with the examination content. Certifying bodies typically provide a content map or outline of areas covered in the test.
- Conduct a self-assessment. "In which areas do I have a strong knowledge base? In what areas am I most comfortable? In what areas do I need to learn more?" (Fights, 2015). Check for tools provided in review books or certifying body's website resources.
- Organize your priorities based on your identified study needs. You can request to be assigned to patients or an area to broaden your knowledge.
- Review the reference list provided in study materials. Take time to read the high priority areas using the references given.
- Check on the required application or testing fee involved.

Table 7.3

Examples of Eligibility Requirements for Certification				
Certification (Certifying Body)	Education	Number of Practice Hours Needed to Apply	Type of Experience	Contact Hours
Certified Pediatric Nursing (Pediatric Nursing Certification Board)		1,800 in the past 24 months *or* A minimum of 5 years as an RN in pediatric nursing *and* 3,000 hours in pediatric nursing within the last 5 years with a minimum of 1,000 hours within the past 24 months	Clinical, management, education, consultation	None
Professional Development (American Nurses Credentialing Center [ANCC])	Bachelor's or higher degree in nursing	Have practiced the equivalent of 2 years full-time as an RN	Have practiced the equivalent of 2 years full-time as an RN; have a minimum of 4,000 hours of clinical practice in nursing professional development within the last 5 years	Have completed 30 hours of continuing education in nursing professional development within the last 3 years

General Test-Taking Strategies

Before the Test

- Enroll in a review course that specialty nursing organizations either sponsor or endorse. See what works best for you: face-to-face, online, audio, or a combination of these modalities. Provide time for self-study after you complete the review course.
- Practice, practice, practice.

During the Test

Test-taking strategies (ANCC, 2019)

- Look for key points in the question such as age, medical diagnosis, time frame, comorbidity.

- Look for key words such as *except, always, first, best.*
- Thoroughly read each question, and answer it, before looking at choices.
- Conserve mental energy.
- Never assume information that is not given.
- All information needed to answer the questions is provided.
- There are 25 questions that are ungraded.
- Answer the easy questions first; mark and return to the difficult questions later.
- Answer *all* questions.

Maintaining Your Certification

Specialty nursing certifications need to be renewed every 3 to 5 years. Recertification requires submission of application for renewal, completion of continuing education hours, and payment of a recertification fee. Nurses renewing their certification are also required to abide by the standards of conduct outlined by the certifying body. Failure to comply with these rules may forfeit eligibility for renewal.

Barriers to Being Certified

Nurses have identified barriers to being certified, including not having enough time to prepare for the exam, the cost of the exam, test-taking anxiety, lack of employer rewards, fear of failure, and cost of the continuing education needed to maintain certification (Garrison, Schulz, Nelson, & Lindquist, 2018).

Not Having Enough Time to Prepare for the Exam

Preparing for the exam requires time and commitment. A typical exam has 175 to 225 test items, covering multiple content areas. I recall preparing and taking the test several years back. A colleague who just sat down for the test at that time shared her review materials with me. One book covered the concepts included for the specialty area. In my case, it was nursing professional development. Another book was in question-and-answer format. These two materials combined came to over 300 pages. I also had to supplement my preparation with other materials such as quality and safety sources online. I gave myself about 60 days to prepare for the test. Don't count on that timeline, as this really depends on your level of preparation. Others may need less or more time than that.

Cost

Check with your institution for any available financial support for certification. Some institutions have a reimbursement program for the certification examination fee or certification renewal fee. Some certifying bodies also offer group discount programs, backed with an agreement with employers. One program provides a discount code to the organization after an agreement is signed. The organization gives the discount code to their nurses who are applying to take the certification test. Each nurse is given two opportunities to pass the test. The organization only gets billed if the nurse successfully passes the test. Other certifying bodies offer certification vouchers at bulk pricing, also through the employers. Certification vouchers are issued directly by the employers for their nurses to use when applying for the certification test.

Test-Taking Anxiety

Feelings of test-taking anxiety can be worse for some nurses than others. The anxiety may evolve from the fear of failing the exam. It is helpful to have conversations with colleagues who just successfully took the test. They will usually be quick to offer you reassurance and a realistic perspective on what to expect on the exam.

Lack of Employer Rewards

Employer support can come in the form of financial support covering the testing fee or free test preparation courses. In addition, some organizations offer a certification bonus to newly certified nurses. Lack of these incentives may be perceived as a barrier by some nurses.

Fear of Failure

Studies have shown that nurses tend to have higher test anxiety level than the average person (35% compared to 16%–20%). Fear of failure can hold you back from pursuing your certification test (www.cpancapa.org). To overcome this fear, experts recommend adequate preparation, strong organization, and proper practice. These strategies allow you to have better control of your fear of the unknown.

Cost of Continuing Education Needed to Take the Certification Test

The cost to take a certification test can range from $2,000 to $3,000, which includes testing fees and review preparation classes. On top of that, you need to complete continuing education to be eligible for the test. The cost associated with this step can be a barrier for some nurses. Free opportunities are available online and through your own organization. Inquire from your department of nursing professional development for resources. If you are a member of a professional nursing organization, continuing education programs are also offered for free or at a lower cost throughout the year.

BECOMING AN EXPERT THROUGH CONTINUING EDUCATION

Training Programs

You can be an expert through training programs. Here are some roles that can be achieved through alignment of experience, interest, and continuing education.

- Lactation consultant
- Patient safety specialist
- Nursing documentation specialist
- Certified wound ostomy nurse

Special Roles

Through the course of your career, opportunities may come for special roles, interim roles, or additional roles for you. Carefully consider how these could present a meaningful experience for you and build your credentials and expertise. I have seen many senior nurses on the unit being invited to be in an interim nurse manager role when a manager goes on leave. I have also seen many of them assume those roles permanently. Nurses who are asked to be in electronic documentation committees may also see leadership positions in informatics come up.

MY JOURNEY TO ACADEMIC PROGRESSION AND BECOMING AN EXPERT

As a new immigrant here in the United States over a decade ago, I had to restart my nursing career, including taking the NCLEX® and starting with an entry-level nursing position in a medical-surgical unit. I completed my master's education in the Philippines and was in the middle of my PhD program when my family and I moved to the United States.

Education

I worked as a clinical practice nurse in the Division of Gastroenterology and Hepatology at the Hospital of the University of Pennsylvania. During my orientation class when I was hired, I learned that the hospital offered an excellent tuition benefit. The hospital would pay for 100% of the tuition fee up front. Being a new immigrant, I had no idea how expensive it was to go to school in the United States. To be eligible, I needed to have worked for at least 6 months at the hospital. Having worked in academia before we moved, I was very motivated to continue further education. My master's degree was focused on nursing education with a concentration in maternal-child health. For my master's research project, I determined the survival rate of low birth weight babies. As a novice researcher, I found it very rewarding to be able to contribute to the knowledge of caring for such a vulnerable population of infants. It was a very positive experience for me and is one aspect of my early nursing career that I would love to re-experience.

After my orientation period, I started looking for an educational program to pursue. I learned of a post-master's certificate in nursing education at the University of Pennsylvania School of Nursing. I inquired about the program, set up a meeting with one of the program advisers, and decided that it was a great program for me. I applied to the program, got accepted, and found myself back in school in a foreign country that fall. It felt overwhelming in the beginning, especially being in a new country and just having transitioned into the workforce. However, I also quickly realized that every student in the class was facing some form of unique challenge—whether it was having a new baby, living far away with a long commute, or aging parents. The school is committed to the success of its students. I took advantage of this supportive environment and embraced every resource I could get my hands on. Looking back, pursuing further education was one of the best decisions that I have made after relaunching my career here. Going back to school, establishing a nurturing relationship with my professors, and getting to know my classmates who came from diverse settings of nursing was just the beginning of my narrative on how I expanded my professional network.

After my post-master's certificate, I did not stop. I went on to pursue my DNP degree at The Johns Hopkins University. For my DNP project, I developed and tested a nurse-driven pathway in hepatitis C management. I implemented this right in my hospital. I am incredibly grateful to have been surrounded by a highly supportive team and some of the best minds in gastroenterology medicine and nursing. After graduation, I submitted several abstracts for presentation at the Society of Gastroenterology Nurses and Associates (SGNA) annual course. All abstracts were accepted as either a poster or podium presentation. One of the abstracts I submitted was on "Everything You Need to Know About Hepatitis C: A Step-by-Step Guide for the GI Nurse." This turned out to be an annual offering at the conference for several years. This opened up many opportunities for me to share and speak about my work in hepatitis C and the liver. I was invited to be a member of the SGNA Research Committee, charged with developing and implementing the research agenda at the national level. The following year, I became part of the SGNA Education Committee and now currently chair this committee. Going back a decade ago when I started my career here in the United States, I would have never thought that I would be leading in this capacity at the national level.

CONCLUSION

When you are beginning your nursing career, you are eager to start your first job. As soon as that happens, it is easy to get caught in the comfort of a familiar routine and to put professional development as a secondary priority. You will get constant reminders and advice about professional development from your manager and peers, or you could even be prompted by your board of nursing when you renew your nursing license.

Key Points

- Keep learning. Keep growing. Aim to be an expert in your specialty.
- Becoming an expert takes time, hard work, and involves a personal strategic plan.
- Pursuing certification, advanced training, or an advanced degree is a way to advance in the field and become an expert.

References

American Academy of Colleges of Nursing. (2019). *DNP fact sheet*. Retrieved from https://www.aacnnursing.org/News-Information/Fact-Sheets/DNP-Fact-Sheet

American Nurses Credentialing Center. (2019). *How to prepare for ANCC exams*. Retrieved from https://www.nursingworld.org/~49e2eb/globalassets/certification/success-pays/test-taking-tips.pdf

Competency and Credentialing Institute. (2019). *Why certify*. Retrieved from https://www.cc-institute.org/why-certify/

Fights, S. (2015). Reap the benefits of certification. *Journal of Trauma Nurses, 22*(1), 3–4. doi:10.1097/jtn.0000000000000105

Garrison, E., Schulz, C., Nelson, C., & Lindquist, C. (2018). Specialty certification: Nurses' perceived values and barriers. *Nursing Management, 49*(5), 42–47. doi:10.1097/01.NUMA.0000532328.69992.fc

Hagan, J., & Curtis, D. L., Sr. (2018). Predictors of nurse practitioner retention. *Journal of the American Association of Nurse Practitioners, 30*(5), 280–284. doi:10.1097/JXX.0000000000000049

Haskins, M., Hnatiuk, C. N., & Yoder, L. H. (2011). Medical-surgical nurses' perceived value of certification study. *Medsurg Nursing, 20*(2), 71–77, 93.

Health Resources and Services Administration. (2019). *Advanced nursing education workforce (ANEW)*. Retrieved from https://www.hrsa.gov/grants/find-funding/hrsa-19-003

Horn, K., Pilkington, L., & Hooten, P. (2019). Pediatric staff nurses' conceptualizations of professional development. *Journal of Pediatric Nursing, 45*, 51–56. doi:10.1016/j.pedn.2019.01.002

Institute of Medicine. (2011). *The future of nursing: Leading change, advancing health*. Washington, DC: The National Academies Press. doi:10.17226/12956

Leonardi, B. (2011). *The value of specialty certifications*. Retrieved from https://www.travelnursing.com/news/features-and-profiles/the-value -of-specialty-certifications/

Lesh, A. T. (2016). *RN to BSN programs benefit nurses and healthcare*. Retrieved from https://www.nurse.com/blog/2016/09/01/rn-to-bsn -programs-benefit-nurses-and-healthcare/

McComas, P. (2011). Practicing to potential. *Johns Hopkins Nursing*. Retrieved from https://magazine.nursing.jhu.edu/2011/12/practicing-to-potential/

New York State Senate. (2017). *Senate Bill S6768*. Retrieved from https:// www.nysenate.gov/legislation/bills/2017/s6768

nursejournal.org. (2020). *25 Reasons why to get a masters in nursing*. Retrieved from https://nursejournal.org/msn-degree/25-best-reasons -why-to-get-a-msn-degree/

Prafder, E. (2017). *Weight the costs and values of a master's degree*. Retrieved from https://nypost.com/2017/06/05/weigh-the-costs-and-values -of-undertaking-a-masters-degree/

Roberts, D. (2017). What's the benefit of certification? *National Association of Orthopaedic Nursing, 36*(6), 377–378. doi:10.1097/NOR.00000 00000000405

Todd, E. M., Watts, L. L., Mulhearn, T. J., Torrence, B. S., Turner, M. R., Connelly, S., & Mumford, M. D.. (2017). A meta-analytic comparison of face-to-face and online delivery in ethics instructions: The case for a hybrid approach. *Science, Engineering, Ethics, 23*, 1719–1754. doi:10.1007/ s11948-017-9869-3

8

Embracing a New Culture

Uvannie Enriquez

"You will meet a lot of barriers that can easily erode your confidence. You have to be resilient."

—Rita K. Adeniran, DrNP, RN, NEA-BC, FNAP, FAAN

The U.S. Bureau of Labor Statistics (BLS) deemed the job outlook for nurses as promising. While the average growth for all occupations within the U.S. economy is projected to be about 5%, the employment growth for RNs is predicted to be significantly higher at 12% by 2028 (BLS, 2019). This translates to substantial employment prospects for internationally educated nurses (IENs) who comprise 15% of all RNs in the United States (George Mason University, Institute for Immigration Research and the Immigrant Learning Center, 2016). The globalization of nursing over the last 50 years enabled foreign nurses to migrate and mitigate the U.S. nursing shortage. If you look around your workplace, you will most likely see at least one IEN or nurse immigrant. Have you ever wondered how they transition into a new country as a nursing professional or how they learn and adapt to a new culture? This chapter focuses on IENs and nurse immigrants, and provides insights on their transition as new nurses in a foreign country, including the unique challenges they encounter and inspiring stories on how they overcome them.

THE TRANSITION PROCESS AS A NEW NURSE IMMIGRANT

Visa Application and Processing

The International Council of Nurses (ICN) ascertained the primary reasons nurses migrate as "improved learning and practice opportunities, better quality of life, pay and working conditions, and personal safety" (ICN, 2010). Unfortunately, nurse migration is complex, arduous, and cost-prohibitive. Despite the looming nursing shortage, immigration continues to slow down due to visa retrogression and other immigration policy shifts. Employment-based green cards are limited only to baccalaureate-prepared IENs. IENs are subjected to multiple rigorous vetting processes, including education eligibility validation, professional licensure status, nursing competency qualification exams, and English language proficiency, before they are able to reside and work in the United States. Although there are other Nursing Commission–approved credentialing companies such as the International Education Research Foundation (IERF) and Educational Records Evaluation Services (ERES), the Commission on Graduates of Foreign Nursing Schools International, Inc. (CGFNS) is the preferred service provider approved by the United States Department of Homeland Security (DHS). The cost of a comprehensive credential evaluation is substantial for IENs coming from developing countries. From my personal experience, the entire process took roughly 2 years. I welcomed the extended processing time, as I was fresh out of nursing school. Also, I needed 2 years of nursing experience in order to be eligible to apply for an occupational visa.

English Language Proficiency

English language proficiency is a requirement for immigration. It is measured by taking a standardized computer- or paper-based test in four formats: reading, writing, listening, and speaking. The two most popular options are TOEFL (Test of English as a Foreign Language) and IELTS (International English Language Testing System). TOEFL is owned by the Educational Testing Service (ETS) while the IELTS is jointly owned by the British Council, IDP: IELTS Australia, and Cambridge English Language Assessment. Both are accepted globally, although most U.S. institutions prefer TOEFL. There are differences in structure, length, and cost between the two tests. It would be prudent for any test-taker to consider these differences before selecting which test to take.

Taking the NCLEX-RN® Examination

Most state nursing regulatory bodies require IENs to go through the certification program offered by CGFNS in order to be eligible to take the NCLEX-RN. It may, therefore, be necessary to take the CGFNS Qualifying Exam as a prerequisite. The CGFNS Qualifying Exam is a multiple-choice exam that assesses nursing knowledge and practice skills. This exam could be used to predict the likelihood IENs will successfully pass the NCLEX-RN in the future. According to the 2019 Quarterly Examination Statistics, over 7,000 IENs successfully passed the NCLEX-RN exam from January to June and are projected to enter the nursing workforce in the United States (NCLEX Statistics, 2019).

After successfully completing the credentials review and passing the requisite exams, IENs must then find a credentialed nursing recruiting agency or U.S.-based employer to initiate the petition for a visa.

There are multiple visa options available for a foreign nurse looking to work in the United States: TN visa, H-1B visa, or an immigrant visa.

TN Visa

The TN nonimmigrant visa permits qualified Canadian and Mexican nationals to seek temporary employment in the United States. The visa is granted for a period of 3 years with the option of extending by increments of 3 years, indefinitely.

General requirements according to the U.S. Citizenship and Immigration Services (USCIS):

- Applicant must be a citizen of Canada or Mexico.
- Applicant's profession qualifies under the regulations.
- The position qualifies under NAFTA (North American Foreign Trade Agreement).
- Applicant has a prearranged full-time or part-time job with a U.S. employer (but not self-employment).
- Applicant has the qualifications required for the profession.

H-1B Visa

The H-1B visa is an option for a nurse with a bachelor's degree or higher who wishes to work in a specialty occupation. The H-1B visa is capped for a period of 3 years with the option of extending for another 3 years. Only 65,000 H-1B visas are issued per fiscal year.

General requirements according to the USCIS:

- Bachelor's or higher degree or its equivalent is normally the minimum entry requirement for the position.
- The degree requirement for the job is common to the industry, or the job is so complex or unique that it can be performed only by an individual with a degree.
- The employer normally requires a degree or its equivalent for the position.

- The nature of the specific duties is so specialized and complex that the knowledge required to perform the duties is usually associated with the attainment of a bachelor's or higher degree.

Immigrant Visa or Green Card

An immigrant visa is for a nurse who plans to live permanently in the United States. After entering the United States on this visa, the nurse will be granted permanent or conditional resident status. The USCIS determines and issues the nurse a permanent resident card, also referred to as a green card, after admission. Nurses are eligible for a green card as a third preference immigrant worker. This is generally considered the most ideal option.

CHALLENGES ENCOUNTERED

The two main challenges that IENs struggle with are cultural dissonance and unfamiliar nursing practice (Viken, Solum, & Lyberg, 2018).

Cultural Dissonance

Cultural dissonance occurs when IENs are in a state of discord when attempting to reconcile their own cultural beliefs and that of the host country. Profound loneliness or alienation, homesickness, perceived discrimination, and communication struggles are all manifestations of cultural dissonance.

Alienation, Loneliness, and Homesickness

IENs often find themselves alienated during the early phase of acculturation (Ea, 2007). Like a fish out of water, IENs, for instance, struggle to navigate through social conversations at work because they are unfamiliar with the topic of the conversation. The natural recourse at this point is to retreat into oneself, thus heightening their feelings of alienation, loneliness, and homesickness. For social beings like us, the power of social capital cannot be overstated. I was presented with the opportunity to migrate to the United States on an employer-sponsored visa because of a prior relationship and the subsequent friendships that formed from it. Being a new immigrant in Texas, I relied heavily on newfound friends and coworkers to survive and thrive. I took up temporary residence at a friend's home until I was able to get an apartment, which was furnished mostly with hand-me-downs. Friends and colleagues drove me around until I was able to lease a car. Coworkers walked me through the inner workings of the local community. I kept myself open to every birthday, anniversary, and holiday celebration until I didn't have the emotional bandwidth left to accommodate profound feelings of isolation and homesickness. Don't get me wrong, every once in a while, homesickness crept up on me, but I never allowed it to get to the point where I considered quitting my job and returning to my native country.

Strategies

- Advocate for a comprehensive assimilation plan that goes beyond orientation to the facility but also informs you on the basic aspects of the U.S. healthcare system, professional stakeholders, the local community and its norms, populations served, and relevant business practices (Sherwood & Shaffer, 2014). If your facility does not have a formalized transition plan, engage your manager, preceptor, or even your entire team on these topics. Be bold and ask for resources.
- Engage in social activities, whether work related or otherwise. This is the best way to expand your support system. Based on a study of over 4,000 respondents, there is an unequivocal "correlation between the size of an immigrant's self-reported social network and his or her likelihood of achieving success" (Bergson-Shilcock & Witte, 2015). The more friends and families you have in your corner, the better off you'll be.
- Explore your new surroundings. Familiarize yourself with key locations within your new community: grocery stores, restaurants, bus stops, shopping malls, schools, libraries, government offices such as the post office, police station, social service offices.
- Seek out home comforts. Whether it's indulging in ethnic food, displaying family mementos, or speaking your native language with a friend from home, home comforts are effective tools to allay homesickness.
- Be realistic with your goals and give yourself time. Acculturation is a process. In Bergson-Shilcock and Witte's study, the respondents who reside in the United States for a minimum of 6 years were found to be more successful.
- Finally, it is okay to be bicultural. You don't have to fully relinquish your deeply rooted cultural heritage in order to acculturate. Some immigrants are able to successfully synthesize their heritage and host cultures, therefore taking dual cultural identities. Some may even argue that in most instances, biculturalism is the most adaptive approach to acculturalization (Schwartz & Unger, 2010).

Discrimination

Racial discrimination, whether real or perceived, is a phenomenon that continues to embattle IENs. Compared to a few decades ago, society in general has evolved to be more inclusive and tolerant. However, subtle and often unintentional discrimination toward IENs continues to persist in the form of racial microaggression and institutional discrimination. Sue (2010, p. 3) defines microaggressive behaviors as "the everyday verbal, nonverbal, and environmental slights, snubs, or insults, whether intentional or unintentional, that communicate hostile, derogatory, or negative messages to target persons based solely upon their marginalized group membership." Racial microaggression may stem from the perceived notion that IENs are lacking in skill and competency or are taking away opportunities that are otherwise available to "locals." I unfortunately had firsthand experience of this rhetoric. A coworker approached me and told me how it is not "fair" that her daughter had to go through a lottery just to get into a nursing school, while I breezed through unabated. Racial microaggression may come from patients as well. Some patients may decline the services of IENs because they are suspicious of IENs' foreign training and education.

In some cases, IENs may experience institutional discrimination. A classic example is the lack of organizational structure and policies to protect IENs against discriminatory language and behaviors. Most academic medical centers may be progressive and thus may have provisions against discrimination of any form. Some healthcare facilities may not be as inclusive. Unfortunately, the political climate is divisive and racially charged now more than ever. Monocultural communities that were previously insulated from foreign migration may not be as welcoming to the influx of immigrants. This brings to mind a profound experience I had 17 years ago as a newly immigrated IEN. On my first day of work, I met the chief nursing officer (CNO) of the hospital who sponsored me. Within minutes into the pleasantries, she commented about how great my English was. This would be the first of many such comments throughout my journey as an immigrant and, ultimately, a naturalized citizen. I was taken aback but frankly didn't feel in the least offended that she was genuinely surprised that I used the idiom "I flew in. . . ." As this was the culmination of a 2-year ordeal and the fulfillment of my dreams, I was happy to be there, happy to start working, and determined to shut down any noise that undermined that. I was then assigned to work in the postanesthesia unit as I had comparable skill set based on the CNO's assessment. The surgical team was extremely welcoming. I was the first Filipino on the team, the third in the entire hospital. Within days, I encountered a certified registered nurse anesthetist (CRNA) who was covertly hostile. He was dismissive when I asked questions. Every time he spoke to me, he would modulate his voice and articulate every single syllable of every single word. It did bother me, but I mentally retreated and stayed far away from him. One day, I brought his patient into the pre-op area where he was waiting. Seeing that his patient didn't have socks on, he immediately yelled at me, "WHERE-ARE-MY-PATIENT'S-SAAAHHH-CKS?" again pronouncing every single syllable in an exaggerated fashion. I looked around and saw faces of patients and colleagues looking at me in disbelief. Thoroughly embarrassed, I excused myself to the bathroom before tears started pouring. I hated him for subjecting me to these experiences, but I mostly hated myself for not standing up to him. After I emerged from the bathroom and regained my composure, a patient's family walked up to me and said, "You are not dumb. He has no right to talk to you like that." The rest of the people in the room echoed the same sentiment, including the charge nurse. She was extremely supportive and addressed the situation with him. She also wrote him up for unprofessional conduct. Through the urging of my manager, I submitted a letter of complaint detailing all the derogatory encounters I had with him. This nurse had multiple prior disciplinary actions. My complaint was the proverbial straw that broke the camel's back. He was ultimately terminated. On his last day, as he walked out of the unit carrying the last of his belongings, he gave me an icy look. To this day, I can still see the hatred in his eyes.

Strategies

- Take a strong stance against normalizing discriminatory language or behavior. The damage of discrimination transcends beyond the intended recipient. Discrimination leads to negative acculturation, stress, and high nurse turnover, which in turn have adverse and insidious effects on nurse–patient ratio, medication errors, and nurse-sensitive quality indicators (Baptiste, 2015).
- Advocate for sensitivity and diversity training and competency for all healthcare staff. The perils of ignorance are profound when it comes to racism.

Communication Struggles

Most newly immigrated IENs struggle with communication. Ironically, after passing the required English test, all immigrants possess some degree of mastery of the English language. However, nuances such as accent, colloquial expressions, and culturally established nonverbal communication are not taught but rather learned through immersion. As an example, while some cultures perceive direct eye contact as disrespectful, the opposite can be said for the American culture. Medical terminology, abbreviations, units of measure, and names of medication and equipment may also differ in the United States. Paracetamol in the United Kingdom and Philippines, for instance, is known as acetaminophen in the United States. IENs must learn to navigate through these variations, especially in the workplace as it largely impacts patient care. Communication, as it pertains to authority structure, also varies from culture to culture. The American culture adopts a more congenial, collaborative, and fluid power structure with a mostly unobstructed bidirectional communication pathway. Some conservative cultures, however, follow a more rigid hierarchy with unyielding respect for authority. Communication largely comes from the top. It was quite an adjustment for me to refer to managers and anyone who was an authority figure by their first names.

Strategies

- Train your ear on the subtleties of the language by watching television shows, listening to the radio (Ea, 2007), and listening intently to conversations. I consider myself to have a good command of American English. In the Philippines, English is the medium of instruction. Classes are taught in English, and all our books are in English, except for the Filipino language course. Although I grew up learning English grammar since pre-K, I mostly attributed my American accent and inflections to all the American shows I watched in the Philippines. I remember reading the newspaper aloud, trying to sound like a CNN newscaster, to the amusement of my sisters.
- Invest in English language training. According to Bergson-Shilcock and Witte (2015), it is "likely the single most powerful step an individual can take toward his or her future employability." In their study, "stronger English language skills were correlated with virtually every possible measure of immigrant economic success."

Unfamiliar Nursing Practice

Nursing, as it is practiced in the United States, can be vastly different from other countries. The delivery of care is mostly patient and family centered. There is a tremendous focus on the patient experience to the point of the government incentivizing positive patient experience. IENs often take on the unfamiliar role of purveyors of customer service, patient educators, independent decision-makers, and bedside leaders. Protocols and intervention bundles may also be unfamiliar to IENs. Unlike some cultures where only the physicians are revered, in the United States, nurses and physicians are on a level playing field. Both are independent in their practice, yet actively collaborating with each other and with the rest of the care team.

Strategies

- Engage in a mentorship program that clarifies roles and maximizes opportunities for patient care, interdisciplinary staff interaction, and skills refinement (Ea, 2007).
- Take an enterprising approach toward professional development by attending continuing education classes, certifying in a

specialized field, or pursuing higher education. Bergson-Shilcock and Witte (2015) concluded that "immigrants who had invested in additional U.S. education were more likely to be successful."

GROWING AS A NURSE IMMIGRANT

The last phase of acculturation is cultural adaptation. Positive acculturation is characterized by the successful reconciliation of the differences between the heritage and host cultures (Ea, 2007). IENs are generally more assertive, driven, and may possess a more passionate outlook on sociopolitical issues. At this stage, the question becomes, "Now what?"

Be a Member of a Professional Organization

Dr. Emerson Ea came to the United States from the Philippines in 1994 on a H-1A visa, a visa specifically available to foreign nurses to temporarily address the nursing shortage at the time. The H-1A nurse program, enacted by the Nursing Relief Act of 1989, expired on September 1, 1995. Within 4 months from visa application, Dr. Ea found himself in New York, ready to start a new life. Within 2 to 3 years, he took advantage of the opportunities in the United States and pursued advanced studies. It didn't take him long to become a member of numerous professional organizations. In 2005, he became the vice president of Lambda Iota, Long Island University School of Nursing's Honor Society. The following year, he became a board member of the Philippine Nurses Association of New York. He also held various posts within Upsilon Chapter, Sigma Theta Tau International, New York University College of Nursing. In 2014, he became a member of the Asian American and Pacific Island Nurses Association. Within the next few years, he became a board member of the Filipino American Human Services (FAHSI), Foundation for Filipino Artists, Inc., and Kaplan Nursing. He is also a task force member of the Quality and Safety Education for Nurses (QSEN) International.

He believes that membership in a professional organization is the best way to network and give back. He also insists on being heard, as opposed to standing in the sideline. This is evident by the many executive positions he held or continues to hold. Dr. Ea is currently the assistant dean for clinical and adjunct affairs at the New York University (NYU) Rory Meyers College of Nursing and was recently inducted as a fellow of the American Academy of Nursing.

Pursue Higher Education

As a new immigrant in the United States over a decade ago, Dr. Rhoda Redulla started with an entry-level nursing position in a medical-surgical unit at the Division of Gastroenterology and Hepatology at the Hospital of the University of Pennsylvania (HUP). She completed her master's education in the Philippines and was in the middle of her PhD program when she and her family moved to the United States. During her orientation class, she learned that the hospital offered an excellent tuition benefit. The hospital would pay 100% of the tuition fee up front. Having worked in academia in the Philippines, she was very motivated to further her education. Her master's degree was focused on nursing education with a concentration in maternal-child health. For her scholarly project, she investigated the survival rate of low birth weight babies. As a novice researcher, she found it very rewarding to be able to contribute to the knowledge of caring for such a vulnerable population of infants.

As an immigrant, she was uncertain if her master's degree in the Philippines would be recognized in the United States. Initially looking for a master's degree, she set up a meeting with an admission officer. She recalled being asked why she was considering another master's degree when she already has one. She then had her educational credentials evaluated by an accredited credentialing agency. As suspected, her foreign degree was deemed equivalent to a master of arts in nursing (MAN) degree in the United States. After confirming this, she decided to pursue a post-master's certificate in nursing education as a way of refresher and to learn more about the educational system in the United States. The following year, after completion of her post-master's certificate, she started applying to doctoral programs. She applied and got accepted to the DNP degree program at Johns Hopkins University.

Dr. Redulla shared that going through the admissions process for an advanced degree was challenging in itself. As a nurse immigrant, you have to go through additional steps to apply. It takes a lot of determination to complete the application process. You have to undergo the credentialing process. This entails making multiple phone calls or, sometimes, having to ask a family or friend in your home country to follow up on your documents that are being verified. All these steps require payment of fees or additional money for correspondence.

Perform Civic Duties: Advocate, Vote, Volunteer

Born in Nigeria and an IEN in the United States, Dr. Rita Adeniran's experiences as a leader, administrator, educator, and professional nurse offer a valuable perspective to anyone interested in improving health and the healthcare system. For example, the Transitioning Internationally Educated Nurses for Success (TIENS) Program that she designed and operationalized at the HUP has been adopted by health systems nationally and globally to help IENs to integrate into host country workforce successfully. The American Nurses Association (ANA) recognized TIENS as a model for integrating IENs into the U.S. workforce in 2008.

Another example is her role as the cochair of the Pennsylvania Action Coalition (PA-AC), Nurse Diversity Council (NDC), from 2013 to 2018. The NDC focuses its work on one of the eight recommendations of the 2010 landmark report by the Institute of Medicine (IOM) and Robert Wood Johnson Foundation (RWJF), *The Future of Nursing: Leading Change, Advancing Health*. The specific suggestion calls for a more diversified and inclusive workforce and underlines the benefit of culturally competent care to optimize health outcomes. Following the IOM report, the RWJF and the American Association of Retired Persons (AARP) partnered and established the Future of Nursing: Campaign for Action to improve the health of all Americans. The campaign is working through national and state level Action Coalitions, engaging with nurses and other stakeholders to advance health and healthcare. The NDC is one of the structures of the PA-AC. Congruent with the strategic goals to build broader coalitions, prioritize diversity, and gather better data to measure gains, the NDC initiated a multiprong strategy to address the issues of diversity and cultural competency in the state of Pennsylvania. Through the support of the NDC, Dr. Adeniran led the completion and analysis of a state-wide survey that determined opportunities for enhancing cultural competence practices in the state of Pennsylvania and guided educational development to improve clinicians' culturally competency skills. Many commend her track record and commitment to echoing the voice of the vulnerable and addressing issues of inequity, inequality, and exclusion in healthcare with grace.

SUCCESS STORY

Rita K. Adeniran, DrNP, RN, NEA-BC, FNAP, FAAN

President and CEO, Innovative and Inclusive Global Solutions, Inc.;
Assistant Clinical Professor, Drexel University, Philadelphia;
Robert Wood Johnson Executive Nurse Fellow (Alumna: 2012 Cohort);
HRET Cultural Competence Leadership Fellow

Dr. Rita K. Adeniran is on a mission to help others move outside of their comfort zone, opening a new window on old assumptions surrounding language differences that sometimes hinder the best outcomes in healthcare. For almost two decades, she has been delivering fearless, authentic presentations, captivating audience attention and interest with her well-crafted opener: "I get excited because this is my passion. If I get on fast-forward mode, just say, 'Rita, stop!'" Dr. Adeniran's clarity, competence, effectiveness, and proven results are not hindered by her native accent.

She captures her audience, orienting them to a topic on diversity and inclusivity, motivating them to listen and request to hear more. The rave reviews that have come to characterize the feedback from her speeches is a validation that diversity in any form is not the issue. Instead, it is the unconscious handling of what each variable of diversity represents within a specific group or society. Dr. Adeniran understands that humans evaluate people unconsciously, and having a different, nondominant accent is likely to rate low in their evaluations. As a profoundly knowledgeable, sophisticated speaker and leader in building teams amid diversity, she strategically empowers her audience to listen authentically, inspiring them to reap the benefits of what diversity offers by igniting their confidence and personal accountability to diversity. Her energy is infectious, and her meaningful commitment to equity and inclusion is felt throughout the room and beyond. Dr. Adeniran seems to live on "fast-forward."

Dr. Adeniran was the director of diversity and inclusion for the University of Pennsylvania Health System, where she provided strategic leadership and direction for diversity, inclusion, and culturally competent healthcare. She served as the global nurse ambassador for Penn Medicine for over a decade. She developed the Global Nurse Program of the HUP and Penn School of Nursing. In 2012, Dr. Adeniran decided to expand her reach by launching her consulting firm, Innovative and Inclusive Global Solutions (IIGS), which supports healthcare organizations and academic institutions to create and sustain an inclusive and high-performing workforce. She is a RWJF Executive Nurse Fellow alumna, a fellow of the American Academy of Nursing, and a Magnet® Recognition Program Appraiser for the American Nurses Credentialing Center. Presently, she is an assistant clinical professor at Drexel University College of Nursing and Health Professions.

Dr. Adeniran embodies the signature traits of an inclusive leader, a much needed and essential leadership quality considering the current racial strife found throughout the country. She strives to recognize the unique contribution of every individual and to create a space in which every contribution is valued. Anyone who has worked closely with Dr. Adeniran can attest to her ability to inspire others to reach within themselves to find excellence. Similarly, anyone who has participated in a conference call facilitated by Dr. Adeniran knows they will need frequent access to their "unmute" button. Her profound respect for others inspires much of her work. For example, in collaboration with six other RWJF Executive Nurse Fellows, Dr. Adeniran designed and launched a Civility Tool-Kit (www.stopbullyingtoolkit.org) to address workplace bullying. She has delivered speeches in more than 22 countries, including commencement and keynote addresses on adversity and diversity. In May 2017, Dr. Adeniran received the 2017 Healthcare Advocate Award from the Pennsylvania Diversity Council and was inducted into the Drexel 100 (Drexel University's Hall of Fame) for making a significant difference in the world, and received the Every Day Nursing Hero Award from the Pittsburgh Black Nurses in Action for outstanding advocacy and mentorship to nurses. Dr. Adeniran has been elected as a Distinguished Fellow of the National Academies of Practice (NAP) in Nursing, a very high honor that acknowledges outstanding achievements.

Dr. Adeniran's Gracious Space philosophy, adapted from the Center for Ethical Leadership, directs us to invite the stranger and embrace learning in public.

> To "invite the stranger" means that we remain open to diverse perspectives to gain clarity of an individual whose background or other quality may be different from our own; it includes echoing the voice of those that would have otherwise be forgotten. To "learn in public" means that we will genuinely listen to new thoughts or conflicting ideas with an openness to change our minds. It involves assuming positive intent, making efforts to be other-oriented, welcoming diverse opinions, and engaging in authentic dialogue.

How did you transition as a new nurse in the United States?

I arrived in the United States in the fall of 1989 as an RN from Nigeria. Like many immigrants, I experienced a profound sense of loss and worked very hard to learn and acculturate to a new culture that is different from what I had always known. I unlearned, relearned, and continuously opened myself to learning at every opportunity. The problems that confronted me as a person and a professional ebbed mostly by being "Black in America," an elusive concept to me at that time, and something that I still struggle to fully comprehend. With limited knowledge of what it means to be "Black" or classified as a minority in the United States, I found myself continually battling stereotypes, inequalities, cultural disenfranchisement, and the stigma that is associated with my native accent.

Nevertheless, I was determined to excel, so I persevered in the face of several adversities. While I did not win every battle, my Christian faith, steadfast belief in the American dream, and the equal protection guaranteed by the U.S. Constitution rekindled my confidence. I was empowered to endure and look forward to the brighter days ahead.

My first encounter with the U.S. healthcare system occurred in a nursing home. I was working as a nursing aide while waiting to take the U.S. RN licensure examination. There, I observed firsthand the "commercialization of care. " I was challenged to precipitously transition my skills from working in a healthcare system where providers, nurses, and aides allocated more of their work hours to care for patients, with a lesser focus on extensive and time-consuming documentation, to a different healthcare system. I quickly learned that the bottom-line factors heavily into how care is structured and delivered within the U.S. healthcare system. There were times I felt displaced, perplexed, and morally distressed, especially when I get criticized for spending too much time with the patients who needed my care. My superiors at the nursing home emphasized the need for me to find alternative ways to get things done and cut down on the time that I spend with each patient providing care. Equipped with my foundational nursing knowledge and skills, I remained resilient and summoned the courage to do things the way I have been educated. I did not give up on the value to treat each patient with dignity, even when it resulted in completing documentation outside of scheduled work hours to avoid reprimands regarding remuneration for additional work hours. I was willing and committed to sacrificing myself and time to ensure each patient under my care received the best care possible. My work ethics, values, and commitment to dignifying anyone under my care spoke volumes about the person that I am and the leader I will become.

Some of the same superiors who resented me for my meticulous way of caring for patients later confessed that I was doing the right thing, but not in the right environment. They lauded my work, raved about my skills, and opened new doors that I walked through. My experience working in the nursing home reiterated the imperative for me to continue to be myself and maintain my values in any circumstance. I would add that it is essential that immigrant nurses remain resilient as they transition to the new country or workplace, and to not listen to the naysayers. Also, always summon the courage to challenge the status quo respectfully, especially when expectations conflict with your moral values and the right thing. These principles were instrumental not only to a successful transition to the U.S. healthcare environment but also to my role as a contributor and recognized leader in the healthcare industry.

What helped you in your transition here in the United States?

The values instilled in me as well as my innate attributes contributed to my successful transition to the United States. To highlight some of these qualities, I would first and foremost underline my passion, which I see as my willingness to suffer for something bigger than myself! I am a passionate nurse, and I view nursing as a privilege to care for humans during their most vulnerable period of life. Other qualities include my principle to be a gracious human being and eagerness to be open, be self-directed, and to always remember to believe in the greater good, even in the face of adversity. I was never afraid to venture out of my comfort zone; neither did I uphold the fear of failing. Indispensable to my accomplishments is the fortune to have had several mentors along the way.

I was born in Nigeria, a patriarchal society that enables men to dominate women by supporting male authority over females. Women are systemically oppressed and suppressed through the country's educational, political, social, and economic structures. Women are viewed as inferior to their male counterparts and expected to be second to men in anything. Women are supposed to be seen, not heard or be assertive. My innate confident attributes led me down a path of adversity, not just for myself, but sometimes extended to my parents. But I was fortunate to have parents who showed me unconditional love and support. My father found a way to empower me within the confines of the culture; I was educated when my education was not supposed to be a priority. I worked very hard in little ways trying to convince my parents, immediate family members, and educational institutions that there is no reason men should be viewed as superior to women, a position that contradicted the law of the land and family beliefs and values. I was ignored and sometimes disciplined for challenging the status quo. At several points in nursing school, my parents were invited to sign reports that I was rebellious when I was only questioning the status quo. For example, my father was once brought in to acknowledge a statement that I refused to yield to the faculty's advice to withdraw my name from a contest for my nursing school presidency against a male nursing colleague for the same position. He eventually lost the election to me because the students voted me as the school's president—an experience that further enhanced my confidence. I did not win all battles, fighting for gender equality. Still, I continued to engage in the war past Nigeria, the country I was born, and now in my adopted country, America!

I believe some of the knowledge gained through various experiences in Nigeria as an innately assertive young woman, passionate nurse advocating for gender equality, unconsciously prepared me for my transition to the United States. I viewed the barriers that I met as a new immigrant as opportunities, which made me more determined, courageous, focused, and resilient. I sought and engaged with role models that I admire to learn from them, and I continuously look for ways to enhance my knowledge through formal and informal learning.

What is your advice to nurse immigrants?

Any new nurse immigrant to the United States should recognize the enormous and life-changing gift the opportunity provides. Despite the initial transitional challenges, I personally feel privileged and honored to be serving as a nursing professional in the United States. My own nursing story is only possible in the United States, and I applaud all nurse leaders before my time and current colleagues for their work to ensure the profession of nursing continues to be recognized for its unique contribution to society. The leaders before me paved the path to practice autonomously and to be successful in the profession that I so much love and adore! While new immigrant nurses will inevitably be confronted with challenges, I would advise them to be resilient, courageous, and focused. Do not allow any problem on the path of your transition to shatter your confidence or derail the vision you have crafted for yourself. It is essential that you work hard and persevere and do your best to turn challenges into opportunities. Do not be afraid to question the status quo, but do so respectfully. It is imperative not to take things personally, and always be gracious and trust enough to be vulnerable. Do your best to assume positive intent; it will save you a lot of unnecessary headaches. Understand that those who may want to exclude you enjoy the luxury of obliviousness. Some exclusionary actions may be done unconsciously, and understand that these individuals may not even know the implications of their exclusionary actions/decisions.

Be strategic when engaging in conversations about politics, any variables of diversity, and marginalization, as these are often emotionally charged topics and can be divisive. People may not forgive your ignorance of the social contexts that these topics operate within the United States because your born country experience may be lacking the historical background, implications, and positions on these issues.

There were things I learned the hard way, but I am very fortunate that I overcame most of them! Do not take words literally; Americans use a lot of slang in communicating and may make gestures to express information that you may receive as a commitment. For example, if a colleague said, "Let's do lunch soon," do not think you will be going out for lunch; it may just be a gesture to express their interest in friendship and getting to know you more! More than anything, be authentic!

I am thankful to God that I was able to navigate the complicated journey of a new nurse immigrant. My gratitude to all my mentors, university professors, and work colleagues who consciously or unconsciously helped me learn the American way. Even as a proud American today, I am still on the journey of learning. Every day, I learn something new.

Key Points

- The process of acculturation is long, complex, and multidimensional.
- IENs are often subjected to unique challenges that test their resilience and grit.
- It is worthwhile to invest in the successful acculturation of IENs as they enrich the U.S. healthcare system and contribute to the delivery of patient care.

References

Baptiste, M. (2015). Workplace discrimination: An additional stressor for internationally educated nurses. *OJIN: The Online Journal of Issues in Nursing, 20*(3). doi:10.3912/OJIN.Vol20No03PPT01

Bergson-Shilcock, A., & Witte, J. (2015). *Steps to success: Integrating immigrant professionals in the U.S.* New York, NY: World Education Services. Retrieved from https://knowledge.wes.org/rs/317-CTM-316/images/Steps_to_Success_WES_IMPRINT_Immigrant_Integration_Survey_United_States-v2.pdf

Bureau of Labor Statistics, U.S. Department of Labor. (2019, September 4). *Occupational outlook handbook: Registered Nurses.* Retrieved from https://www.bls.gov/ooh/healthcare/registered-nurses.htm

Ea, E. (2007). Facilitating acculturation of foreign-educated nurses. *OJIN: Online Journal of Issues in Nursing, 13*(1). doi:10.3912/OJIN.Vol13No01PPT03

George Mason University, Institute for Immigration Research and the Immigrant Learning Center. (2016, June). *Immigrants in health care:*

Keeping Americans healthy through care and innovation. Retrieved from https://www.ilctr.org/wp-content/uploads/2017/09/Immigrants_in _Healthcare_FACT_SHEET.pdf

International Council of Nurses. (2010). *Career moves and migration: Critical questions guidelines*. Retrieved from https://www.icn.ch/sites/default/ files/inline-files/2010_guideline_career_moves_migration_eng.pdf

NCLEX Statistics. (2019). *Quarterly examination statistics*. Retrieved from https://www.ncsbn.org/NCLEX_Stats_2019.pdf

Schwartz, S. J., & Unger, J. B. (2010). Biculturalism and context: What is biculturalism, and when is it adaptive? Commentary on Mistry and Wu. *Human Development, 53*(1), 26–32. doi:10.1159/000268137

Sherwood, G., & Shaffer, F. (2014). The role of internationally educated nurses in a quality, safe workforce. *Nursing Outlook, 62*(1), 46–52. doi:10.1016/j. outlook.2013.11.001

Sue, D. W. (2010). Microaggressions, marginality, and oppression: An introduction. In D. W. Sue (Ed.), *Microaggressions and marginality: Manifestation, dynamics, and impact* (pp. 3–22). Hoboken, NJ: Wiley.

Viken, B., Solum, E. M., & Lyberg, A. (2018). Foreign educated nurses' work experiences and patient safety—A systematic review of qualitative studies. *Nursing Open, 5*(4), 455–468. doi:10.1002/nop2.146

9

Nursing as a Second Career

Peter Stoffan

"If you think that this is the career for you, give your 100%, because the patients deserve nothing less. Nurse with your actions, your mind and your words. They are all powerful ways to help patients."
—Janine Llamzon, MS, AGNPc, RN, CEN, NEA-BC

If you are considering a nursing career or are considering becoming a second-career nurse, this chapter is for you! Inside this chapter, you will find some letters written to prospective, current, and graduated students pursuing nursing. Whether nursing is a second career for you, my hope is you will glean new information or arrive at a fresh perspective that may be beneficial as you continue your amazing career path. This chapter discusses the choice to go back to school and how to choose the right school for you. Other topics covered include how to prepare for the NCLEX-RN® licensure exam and how to prepare for your next phase of life postgraduation. Additionally, you—the reader—will hear from other second-degree nursing students and how they made the schooling and career switch successfully. You will hear how you, as a unique individual, can enhance the discipline of nursing through highlighting what makes you special! How can you bridge the gap between your first- and second-degrees while remaining true to yourself!?

MY STORY

My name is Peter Stoffan. My first degree is a BA in musical theater from Indiana University. I moved to New York City and pursued acting for many years. I always knew I would go back to school, but I didn't know for what. As a "dancer," I realized my hips and knees wouldn't be able to last forever. (Note: *Dancer* is in quotes because though I could high kick and turn just like the rest of my colleagues, part of me always felt like a poser faking my way through a dance class.) Additionally, many of the successful Broadway-credited actors I know go months, and sometimes years, between "big breaks." Therefore, I knew I wanted a solid "back-up plan" that I could rely on and still feel fulfilled.

I thought, perhaps, I would go to school for education to teach theater or get a degree in physical therapy to rely on my movement background. After soul-searching for some time between gigs one winter, I thought about pursuing nursing. My brother Alex and my grandpa Harold are physicians, so I realized healthcare was in my blood. I have a cousin who is a women's health midwife/nurse practitioner, my great-aunt Esteleen is a nurse, and my grandma Sally was a nurse. My grandma Sally died of Parkinson's-related health issues. Watching her die and helping her through that process was inspirational. Many days, I sat with her and helped her with her afternoon medications. Due to her poor motor control, it took her about an hour and a half to swallow her myriad of pills that were to help control her many symptoms. I'll never forget one day sitting on her porch outside and her trying to say "Thank you" for helping with a simple task of swallowing pills and water—I felt a great sense of humility and pride. If I could help others in any way, large or small, I thought how special. I realized the potential a nurse has to make a difference.

I applied to NewYork-Presbyterian Hospital as a unit clerk, and I was happy I was offered the job. Nursing shortages exist in many places, but New York City is not one of them. I knew that I wanted to be competitive once I earned my nursing degree, so being employed at a hospital before I graduated could give me the extra edge I needed in the competitive NYC job market. I didn't waste much time, and once I started the job in the hospital, I started applying to nursing schools.

If I were to become a nurse, I had to get the sciences foundation somehow and somewhere. I enrolled in BMCC (Borough of Manhattan Community College) to complete my prerequisites for nursing school. For second-degree students, most schools require prerequisites before enrolling in an accelerated 12- or 18-month BSN program (see the section "Which School?"). The typical accelerated BSN program is a second-degree program designed for students who already have a baccalaureate degree in a nonnursing major and requires 11 to 18 months of full-time study for degree completion. Accelerated BSN programs build on previous learning experiences and provide a way for individuals with undergraduate degrees in other disciplines to transition into nursing (American Association of Colleges of Nursing [AACN], 2019).

Needless to say, I didn't take the preceding courses while studying musical theater. During my BA degree, I skipped and avoided all the chemistry, biology, and math courses. I would rather jump into the tap dance, Shakespeare acting, costuming, and history of the Roman Spectacle courses any day. I wanted to go somewhere affordable and local, so BMCC was the choice I made. After going to the BMCC registrar's office, many of my required classes were full. It seemed that because I chose an affordable option, competition was higher to enter the classes. I also didn't like the answers, or lack thereof, I was getting from academic advisers at the local and affordable school. It seemed that because I chose an affordable option, the service was less than premier. I immediately started considering other options for school. I started looking at New York University (NYU). Years prior, I applied and auditioned for NYU's musical theater program for my first degree, and I was heartbroken when I didn't get in. Looking back, I loved my time at Indiana University and created many lifelong friendships and received an amazing well-rounded education while receiving world-class vocal training! The chance to go to NYU after all seemed like an amazing opportunity. I applied, and I got in. And then I paid and am still paying, and probably I will continue to pay off my student loans for many years ahead. That said, I received excellent service and never waited to enter a class. I did something stupid, though. I took my prerequisites at NYU, which means I took an entire year of courses at the NYU price prior to entering the 15-month accelerated program. Taking the prerequisites at NYU was not an intelligent economical decision, but it made my transition from prerequisites to nursing core classes much easier.

The accelerated program was designed to work for a working professional like me. I had a goal in sight, and I was happy the timeline was preset. It kept me focused. Four semesters straight through was very manageable for me because I did not have a full-time job. Once the true accelerated program began, I switched my position from a full-time unit clerk to a per diem nurse companion. As a nurse companion, I could work a few 12-hour shifts a month, sitting with patients who were delirious or needed 1:1 supervision. The main objective was to gain additional clinical experience while remaining on the hospital payroll so once I graduated I could just "transfer" to a nursing position instead of applying as a new candidate. I had a few colleagues who were working full-time or part-time through the accelerated program, and they still managed to get through the degree but perhaps with a bit more stress and a bit less sleep. Most schools do not suggest working through an accelerated program because of the full-time class requirement in addition to the nursing clinical component. My advice to anyone would be to listen to yourself and balance your own needs with the school requirements. While you want to get the most out of the degree program, people also need to support themselves and their families, so balance school with your life thoughtfully.

I am forever proud of myself for deciding to go back to school for nursing, and I know you will be, too.

ADVICE FOR NURSES THINKING OF PURSUING NURSING AS A SECOND CAREER

Here I have written some letters to people who are considering, are pursuing, or have earned a second degree in nursing. These letters reflect my heartfelt advice and aim to pose and answer questions, highlight successes and pitfalls, and stimulate thought. I am happy to share my personal experience, including the fears and joys of redirecting a life and career. I hope sharing my vision, story, experiences (personal and shared), and reflections can help you in some way.

For Those Considering a Second Degree in Nursing

Dear Brave Ones,

First, congratulations! You are thinking about doing something major and drastic to change your life. Making this decision is a big one, and you should not take it lightly. I have some questions for you:

- Why are you choosing to go back to school?
- Why are you choosing nursing?
- What school(s) are you considering, and why?
- What kind of nurse do you want to be?

I applaud you for taking this leap. I know you will be able to draw upon your first degree and your inherent talents and skills to make you a more accomplished and successful nurse. Please read the rest of this chapter, as I hope to go over some important highlights of this next phase of your life. I also plan to give any advice if I had the chance to do it again!

Respectfully Admiring Your Bravery,

PS

For Those Already Pursuing a Second Degree in Nursing

Dear Students,

Way to go! You are doing it, one care plan at a time. Don't worry, nursing isn't all care plans (but sometimes you wish it would be!). And yes, care plans are important. They help synthesize and put down on paper that each patient requires a complete understanding of the many comorbidities, diagnosed and undiagnosed, to effectively take care of and manage the person as a whole. Nursing school doesn't last forever, so I challenge you to soak it all up and enjoy as much as possible!

So you are in nursing school, and the end is in sight. But what's next? Some questions for you:

- Have you thought about what type of nurse you want to be? How will you know to find the best fit?
- How is your résumé looking? Are you ready to look for jobs?
- How will you use your skills from your first degree or "first life" to enhance your nursing career?

If you are in school full-time without working, definitely enjoy the time you have to focus on your schooling. If you are in school while working, incredible! Not an easy feat and believe me, it is worth it. Don't stop either way. You can do it. I hope to answer some of the questions I'm asking you and share some success stories and reflections to create a bigger picture for life outside of nursing school.

With Admiration and Cheerleading,
PS

For Those Who Have Already Earned a Second Degree in Nursing

Dear Nurses,

Congratulations. We are forever connected as members of one of the most special and important societies—we are nurses. Did you know that nurses are among the most trusted in the nation/world? Amazing. So, you have the degree, you may already have a job, or you may be reading this years after achieving this degree and most likely a nursing license. Well, have you considered the following questions?

- If you haven't taken the NCLEX-RN licensure exam yet, how are you preparing?
- Are you making the most of your career switch? How will you know?

- Did you waste your time in changing careers?
- What is next? Are you making the most of your nursing career? How are you enhancing the discipline of nursing?

If the preceding questions sparked an internal conflict of knowing the answers or wanting to find the answers somewhere, this chapter will spark some thought and debate as you continue your quest to be the most and best you can be.

Your Nursing Partner,

PS

WHY GO BACK TO SCHOOL?

Why not? The end.

Just kidding. School is something you should embark on only after much thought. School is never easy and should be pursued after weighing all the options you have. Do you want to go to school now, or do you want to wait to go back to school later when you "have more time"? So what are the options you may need to weigh to decide?

Now or later?

I know many second-degree students who have a family and are amazingly successful at balancing work, school, and life. I'm not saying it is easy, but there are many options for second-degree students raising and/or supporting families. A question I know some colleagues have asked themselves prior to starting school is, Will school be easier now or later? (Hint: The answer is usually "now.") As we get older, we won't want to use our energy, time, and resources on school. Also the answer is usually "now" because we will never be closer to finishing our first degree than we are right now! Therefore, we know the tricks and shortcuts to being successful in school. Technology is so entwined with how education is delivered. What will technology look like years from now? Do you want to wait to be behind the curve with technology before you enroll in a second degree? Or do you want to be more aware of the systems and methods used so at least you aren't learning a new software system or delivery method while learning an entire new course of study?

TESTIMONIAL STORY OF SCHOOL AND FAMILY BALANCE

From a second-degree nurse colleague:

"My daughter was 2 years old when I entered into an accelerated nursing program. It was incredibly challenging juggling the needs of my daughter, husband, and household while struggling through a 15-month program in a profession completely new to me. There were a lot of sleepless nights, tears, and anger during those months, but I was able to graduate with honors and won an award for outstanding work in the clinical setting. Looking back, having a child while in school made me stay incredibly organized. It also forced me to take a break from studying every day to spend time with my family. I think these factors helped me succeed. If given the opportunity, I would not go back and change my situation for anything!"

Cost

Cost of study is a major factor when deciding when/where/how to back to school. It is important to get all the facts before enrolling in school. When looking at which school you will be achieving your second degree, make sure to set up appointments with the financial adviser and program director for the school. You can even email or set up a phone call with the individual parties. Getting all the information is paramount to ensure you will not regret your big decision later.

 REFLECTION

If I were to go back and do it again, I would get my prerequisites online or anywhere affordable and then apply as an accelerated program student.

WHY NURSING? WHAT CAN YOU DO WITH A NURSING DEGREE?

Becoming a nurse is amazing. Nurses can do anything. Make sure you are not entering nursing for the money. If you are, you are making the wrong choice. Some states pay very well and respectfully for nurses, but money is never the reason to do anything. We all know the difference of someone who is in a job because of the money and someone who is in the job because they love it.

- Remember that teacher you had who was just downright mean and nasty? I suspect they went into teaching because of the money and probably because a general studies degree didn't automatically give them a job postgraduation.
- Now remember that teacher you had who was inspirational and motivating? I suspect they went into teaching because they loved being able to foster and grow others to the best of their abilities.

Be the good teacher. Become a nurse because you want to help others.
The money in nursing will *never* outweigh the stress, nonsense, emotional frustration, and heartbreak that you may feel during your time in this discipline.

WHICH SCHOOL?

Choosing the right school is important. Remember my story about BMCC and NYU? I chose NYU because it was the right fit for me. I wanted service and expedited entry to classes. I also wanted the name of NYU on my diploma because for me, that is important. I wanted the wall of diplomas with names people all over the globe would recognize. That may not matter to you. You may want to go to the cheapest and quickest school, and that is okay. There are no rules and no guidelines for where to go to school. You need to feel proud and satisfied with whatever decision you make. Do as many Internet searches as possible to find what schools exist. Think about online or in-person learning. What makes the most sense for you? Think about cost. Which schools give scholarships? Does your employer have a tuition reimbursement program? If so, is there a limit, or are there limitations? Think about timing of the classes. Do they offer full-time or part-time learning structures? Never stop asking questions. If you do the preliminary work before enrolling, you will feel satisfied with where you are going to school.

If you are considering applying to a second-degree accelerated nursing program, most schools require prerequisites.

Most schools prerequisites include:

- Anatomy and physiology I and II (two semesters typically)
- Psychology or developmental psychology
- Biochemistry
- Microbiology
- Statistics
- Nutrition

WHAT TYPE OF NURSE DO YOU WANT TO BE?

You may be nearing the end of your degree program, so what are you thinking? Do you have an idea of where you want to work? That is great! However, I challenge you to be flexible with your thinking and not box yourself in to one field or subspecialty. Some specialties such as labor and delivery, pediatrics, operating room, and oncology are amazing and ever-growing and ever-important fields. Because they are specialty fields, however, the nurses I know who have started there often feel "trapped." *This does not have to be the case.* Don't be afraid to start wherever you want and/or wherever you get a job! The best part of being a nurse is the flexibility and the ability to always move jobs and learn a new field. Yes, by becoming a subspecialty nurse, you will learn very specific skills, algorithms, cultures, and protocols, but that does not mean you are trapped. You should feel empowered that because you were able to learn a specific knowledge set, you can learn anything. You can transfer your skills and learning abilities to anything. Again, there is no road map or set of guidelines for how to do something. Make your decision for where to work, knowing that it does not have to be permanent. Enjoy nursing and take advantage of your degree and license.

★★ REFLECTION

I started in the surgical step-down unit. I worked there as the unit clerk while getting my prerequisites, so it was a great transition for me. I am so happy I started on this unit because it gave me a set of general skills for critical care surgical patients. I was on the overnight shift, and I didn't mind working overnight. I never had trouble sleeping because I was tired after working the 12-hour shift and came home and passed out! (I think having blackout shades and an interior-facing bedroom window helped.) I worked on the surgical step-down unit for almost 2 years and transferred to the general surgery postanesthesia care unit (PACU). I loved the PACU because it took the skills I learned from taking care of the postsurgery patients on the step-down unit and allowed me to apply them in a focused way. I never wanted to do anything too specific such as labor and delivery or the operating room, but I applaud those who do!

ARE YOU READY FOR GRADUATION?

If you haven't graduated yet, are you ready? How is your résumé looking? Make sure that when interviewing and building your résumé, you highlight the things that make you the shining individual you are. Nursing is your second degree, so make sure you have things on your résumé that reflect your "first life." As an employer, I want to know what makes you *you!* Previous work experience is incredible on a résumé, especially if it is your first nursing job. If you worked in a restaurant, that's valuable because you can talk about customer service. If you worked in a nonprofit, that's valuable because you know how to navigate work environments and public systems. If you never worked, that's okay, too. Do you have volunteer experience? Do you have tutoring experience? Make sure to put down on paper the best pieces of you. Remember you will be screened for interviews based on that one 8.5-by-11-inch résumé, so make it shine.

When you interview, make sure to be prepared to discuss why you went into nursing. Have your elevator speech ready, but keep it genuine. Also, be prepared to discuss how you will be able to use the skills and knowledge gained from your first degree to make you the best nurse possible. After all, isn't that the point? You don't want the time and money spent for your first degree to be for nothing!

Where are you applying? If you already have a job in a health-care facility, chances are you have a good chance of working there, so good job! If not, that's okay. How do you find the best place to work without knowing the company? Do another Internet search review of the top hospitals. *U.S. News and World Report* has annual reports for the best hospitals. The American Nurses' Credentialing Center also is a good resource for which hospitals have Magnet' status. Magnet designation is the highest recognition of nursing excellence. Magnet-recognized hospitals tend to attract top talent and are known for their excellent practice environment (ANCC, n.d.). Make sure that wherever you are applying, you cast a wide net and remain open to opportunities. It can sometimes be hard to land your first job as a nurse. Stay positive and remain diligent!

★★ REFLECTION

In my experience, people talk about a nursing shortage, but that only seems to be the case in non-urban areas. I know hospitals in urban areas with waitlists of over 500 for nursing candidates! I also know that there are job fairs in non-urban areas looking specifically for nurses. I also know that in a non-urban hospital, the percentage of BSN-prepared nurses is drastically lower than urban hospitals. Competition doesn't exist the farther you go out of any city. Keep that in mind while looking for jobs. Relocation or casting a wider geographical net while applying for jobs may be a good idea.

GETTING THE RN LICENSE AND WHAT TO DO NEXT

You are studying for the NCLEX-RN license. This could be a scary time, but it doesn't have to be. Whatever method you are using, be diligent.

★★ REFLECTION

I used Kaplan's NCLEX prep; it was built into my NYU tuition. Therefore, it was already paid for. I registered for my exam date to be 3 months after graduation, so I had time to celebrate and relax after achieving my BSN and then had time to hunker down and study. I did some basic test preparation, including reviewing and studying the outline of the exam, categories of questions, and how to study. I then reviewed questions daily. I found that I was more focused if I studied outside of my home, so I went to the New York Public Library to review questions. This was an amazing place to study for me because I loved making my studying "an event." It made me feel like I did something other than studying that day. If I felt antsy or not focused and wanted to walk around, I did and then found a new corner of a quiet room to review more questions. I probably started averaging around 25 questions a day (including review of any concepts I didn't feel secure about). One month leading up to the test, I increased to 50 questions a day. A few days I tested myself and would make myself do at least 100 to 150 questions a day so I felt prepared sitting down for that long of a time and remembering concepts in a long stretch. The NCLEX is a test that shuts off after 75 questions if you are either doing well or definitely failing. The test can continue up to 300 questions to validate that you either know the concepts or do not. On test day, I felt very prepared. The test shut off after 75 questions. I panicked. Three days later I received my notice that I passed. I cried. I celebrated with friends. That memory is still very present in my brain and always will be.

MAKING THE MOST OF YOUR CAREER SWITCH

Are you making the most of your career switch? How will you know? I don't think one will ever know if they are "making the most" out of anything. I do think that simply asking if you are "making the most" out of your career is the first step to ensure you are! Are you taking the knowledge and experience gleaned from your first degree to enhance your career in nursing? People ask me all the time, "Do you miss performing/singing/dancing/acting?" The answer is "Yes!" The second answer, however, is that I get to use my musical theater talents and skills in nursing and management every day. Am I reciting a Shakespeare soliloquy or performing an Italian aria to my patients and colleagues? Maybe not. But am I able to relate to people on a different level? Yes. Am I able to perform for patients by putting on a happy face and putting their needs 100% above and before mine? Absolutely.

How can you take what you learned in your previous life experiences and degrees and use it toward your nursing career? If your first degree is in psychology, maybe you can evaluate research studies easier than your colleagues. If your first degree is in English, perhaps you can use your talents to write nursing publications and delineate your unit's performance improvement initiatives. If your first degree is in woodworking, then you have the skills to create something that could benefit your patients and unit. The point is, you can make the most of your nursing career by relying on your entire self, and that includes every ounce of knowledge and life experience you have before and after your second degree.

HOW ARE YOU ENHANCING THE DISCIPLINE OF NURSING?

Okay, so now what? How can you drive the discipline of nursing forward? Never stop questioning. Rely on the talents and skills you have developed your entire life. Nursing is fluid and dynamic, and it needs fluid and dynamic professionals to ensure it is continuously catapulted forward. Go back to school! Get a master's degree. Take your knowledge and skills learned on your unit and solve the problems you see. Healthcare will forever be a saturated and convoluted industry, so it needs problem-solvers.

SUCCESS STORY

Janine Llamzon, MS, AGNPc, RN, CEN, NEA-BC
Director of Clinical Nursing and Operations: Emergency Serviceline, St. Joseph's Health, Paterson

"I never wanted to be a nurse. I lived in the Philippines 27 years of my life. I was not the best student, not because of lack of support or skill, but unwillingness to work harder and sheer preoccupation to the unnecessary. I grew up in a very sheltered environment. My parents worked hard to ensure that they were able to provide me with the best education. I didn't try to have high grades. I thought that passing the school year was good enough.

Then it was time to apply for college. My parents begged me to apply to nursing school. I was adamant about my refusal. Secretly, I wanted to be in advertising. I thought that was 'the dream.' I wanted to work in a multinational advertising firm and help create the best advertising and marketing campaigns that ensured brand success. My parents gifted me a United States vacation prior to starting my first year in college, to dissuade me from advertising and to show me how nurses successfully lived in America. I wouldn't have it. I enjoyed Disneyland, Six Flags, and eating the best steak, but I did not say 'yes' to nursing school.

After failing multiple college applications, I enrolled in an advertising school. I promised myself that I will do better this time. I has on the 'Honor's list.' I graduated with flying colors, and my final scholarly project won the first prize. I interned in the number one advertising agency in the Philippines and was offered a job to join the team that handled their biggest client. I redeemed myself (so I thought).

I got pregnant out of wedlock less than a year of employment. I failed again. Now, I have to pack my bags, go back to my parents' home, and leave advertising behind. My parents talked to me and told me that since I will become a single mother, I needed to make a decision that will make me financially stable to take care of my son.

My life was over.

The years spent in nursing school were a blur. Honestly, I may have been a little depressed at that time. I was in a town I didn't like, I was pursuing a career I didn't want, and I had a child I was not ready for. Little did I know I will be living the best life I have ever had and being the best version of myself.

I left for the United States right after passing the board exam. I was employed in a trauma center in the South Bronx and worked in the emergency department of the poorest zip code in the United States. I felt fire in my heart that I have never felt before. I asked myself, 'Why did I ever resist this?' I felt fulfillment that I have never felt before by being in community with the patients, teamwork among my peers, and creating a safe environment to the underserved.

Purpose.

I became a charge nurse within 3 years, then a nurse manager, then the director of the emergency department—all within 10 years of employment in St. Barnabas Hospital. I studied to become a nurse practitioner, initially to improve my knowledge and skill—but later finding that the reason I want to be a better nurse was to help in the drive to uphold the 'future of nursing and nurses.'

I was the first nurse from St. Barnabas to join the Clinical Quality Fellowship Program by the United Hospital Fund and Greater New York. I was the keynote graduation speaker of the fellowship. I took a chance to be a faculty to the program. Then, the Mount Sinai Hospital Emergency Department offered me a position as the quality program manager of the emergency department. I became Novice Nurse of the Year after a year of employment in St. Barnabas, Nurse Leader of the Year 8 years after, and nurse leader red carpet awardee after a year of employment in Mount Sinai.

Yes, after I resisted so many years, nursing gave me my purpose.

Now, I live the values of nursing in my daily life—compassion, integrity, dignity, justice, and empowerment. I use it in the way I take care of my children. I use it in helping my church community. I use it at work when as we pursue high-reliability and safe, efficient, quality care.

I am now enrolled in a doctor of nursing practice (DNP) program. Why study for the DNP? Because it is my obligation to the future of nursing.

I am passionate about nursing, and I think that it is my responsibility to better myself, to educate myself so that I can influence others to work in the full capacity of their profession.

We are leaders. Nurses are one of the most influential voices in healthcare."

Janine's advice for second-degree nurses

"In my experience, the main drivers of choosing nursing were financial need and the fastest way to create a stable life for my son. Little did I know that those will be the least of the factors that will give me fulfillment. Nursing is not for everyone. When I pursued nursing in 2004, there was a surplus of nursing students. Nursing is not for everyone. Skill, technique, and knowledge are easy to learn and, with practice, can be mastered. However, empathy, integrity, and compassion—which I feel are the main values that separate nursing from other healthcare practitioners—are values that you cannot fake.

1. Reflect. Be honest with yourself if nursing is really for you. If not, it is okay, because there are other fields that you can do.
2. If you think that this is the career for you, give your 100%, because the patients deserve nothing less. Nurse with your actions, your mind, and your words. They are all powerful ways to help patients.
3. Invest in yourself. Don't stop. The nursing profession needs people like you. Going on your second career means that you are willing to do it again, that you don't give up. Keep that fire in you, as the future of nursing relies on people like you.
4. You will settle in. It may take time, but you will get it. Pick role models and mentors. Pick many, and emulate the values and characteristics you feel will make you a better nurse.
5. Have fun. Yes, we work to ensure that we have means to live. Your work family is your family. Have fun with them. Have fun at work. It will make the work less stressful. You will soon realize that your nursing job stops becoming a job and becomes your vocation."

What am I most proud of?

"Just like a whirlwind romance, I was given various opportunities in my nursing career. I had the opportunity to get to know great nursing leaders who have reached out to help me become a better nurse leader. I have the job that I feel I am best at and [in which i can] integrate my first degree. My story epitomizes what I am proud of, but I think the thing that I am most happy about is having the opportunity to teach young nurses.

When I was a staff nurse, I had the opportunity to influence the 20+ patients I had in a day. When I was a nursing director, I have the chance to influence the staff and the 100,000 patients in a year. When I became the quality manager, I am now able to influence the staff, patients, and the future nurses/patients even when I leave Mount Sinai. The quality, safety, and professional practice performance projects that we create change the safety culture of the ED and the other departments that work with us.

This is not just for me but also for the future of nursing and healthcare. I know that I am upholding the future of nursing by being an integral conduit of change and maximizing fully my professional license."

CONCLUSION

The decision to pursue your degree in nursing is only the beginning. Deciding which school and making a commitment to finish your degree is one of the early chapters in your personal nursing journey. What area of specialization will you pick? Work hard and make good connections with those around you, as they will help inform your clinical, professional, and personal decisions. For me, the best thing about being a nurse is that you never stop growing and learning. Nursing is evolving and will need to continue to evolve with the ever-changing healthcare landscape. Taking the leap from your first degree and career to this vital discipline is just the beginning. How exciting!

Key Points

The Author's Hopes

- I hope you feel more proud and excited that you have taken a step to better yourself and the world we live in by becoming a nurse. This choice probably did not come easy and took much balancing of personal, financial, and social needs. Congratulations to you wherever you are in your second-degree journey; taking the leap is always the hardest part!

- I hope you feel confident that there is a place and a path for you. The hard part is knowing that there is no "set path." The path you take will be uniquely yours, and that is okay. I hope this chapter informed you of some pitfalls and successes of other nurses while highlighting that there is no best way to do this amazing career switch. Whatever makes sense to you is what makes sense in the world.

- I hope you feel confident in who you are as an individual and feel confident that your unique traits are the traits that will make you a strong asset to the nursing world. Please don't forget to rely on the education, skills, and talents you have honed over however many years to inform your decisions as a healthcare provider. Your time spent in another degree and/or another career will not be wasted!

References

American Association of Colleges of Nursing. (2019). *Accelerated baccalaureate and master's degree in nursing.* Retrieved from https://www.aacnnursing.org/News-Information/Fact-Sheets/Accelerated-Programs

American Nurses Credentialing Center. (n.d.). *ANCC Magnet Recognition Program*®. Retrieved from https://www.nursingworld.org/organizational-programs/magnet/

J. Llamzon, personal communication, August, 27, 2019.

K. Purrini, personal communication, September, 11, 2019.

WHAT IS NETWORKING?

10

Effective Networking

Lisa Roman-Fischetti

"The word 'networking' meant nothing to me in my years as a bedside nurse. It was a thing business people did; it wasn't relevant for clinicians. Boy, was I mistaken."

—Maureen Mullin, MSN, RN, NEA-BC

When you graduate from a nursing program, you often think, "I did it!" And you're correct. It's a wonderful achievement! You stand at the threshold of a blossoming career. As you begin your journey of growing in expertise and contributing to the health of consumers, opportunities abound. Just say yes! Within your workplace, get involved in structures that support shared decision-making and evidence-based professional practice. Join a professional nursing organization and introduce yourself to members who are part of the broader nursing community.

Share your knowledge and experience. Keep learning and developing your knowledge base through continuing education offerings in your place of practice, through your professional organization, and, when you're ready, through advanced formal education. Be bold! In all of these venues, networking is key to your success. The ability to step out of your comfort zone and make connections can take you farther than you dreamed could happen.

WHAT IS NETWORKING?

Professional networking consists of attempts by individuals to develop and maintain relationships with others who have the potential to assist you in your work or career. Developing and nurturing social bonds with individuals who may provide career assistance serve as an important means of enhancing professional careers. When effective, networking facilitates access to critical career relationships with powerful mentors who could play an important role in your career advancement (Greguletz, Diehl, & Kreutzer, 2019).

Kirsten Drake, DNP, RN (2017), describes three categories of networking: operational, personal, and strategic. Operational networking focuses on getting things done and building relationships with internal organizational contacts. Personal networking focuses on your personal development with contacts outside of your organization. Strategic networking occurs at higher organizational levels and focuses on future priorities, leveraging your internal and external contacts.

Dr. Drake (2017) writes, "Think of networking as relationship building to achieve goals; it isn't just about meeting people. Systematically categorizing your contacts by the type of relationship will help you use them in the future: connectors, mentors, peers, and experts" (p. 56).

Nurse and author Donna Cardillo (n.d.), MA, RN, CSP, FAAN, describes networking as:

> ... very simply, making personal contacts and connections with people. It involves meeting new people and staying in touch with those you already know. Networking is about building relationships. It's a reciprocal process of giving and getting information, advice, and assistance. Networking is done in person, by telephone, by written correspondence, and, now, over the Internet.

KNOWING YOUR STRENGTHS AND LIMITATIONS

The ability to network effectively is important in all professions today. In the nursing profession, you are exposed to skill building in communication and assessment early in your education. Depending on your own personality, you may find it easier or harder to start and maintain a conversation, probe for more information without "grilling" the person you're talking to, and find the right balance between talking and listening. As you grow in these skills, you will benefit personally and professionally. Knowing a bit about your personality type can make networking easier.

Have you taken a personality test as part of your coursework? If you are interested in taking one, there are many free or low-cost options online. Some may even be available through the human resources department at your organization. Many organizations appreciate the value of offering personal and professional development opportunities to their workforce through courses that help individuals to strengthen their work relationships within their team and cross-functionally with other teams. Three well-known examples are DISC Assessment, Myers-Briggs Type Indicator˚ (MBTI˚), and CliftonStrengths.

DISC, created by William Marston (1928), is a behavioral style assessment that can help an individual improve his or her interpersonal communications and work relationships. Discover your DISC style and learn how to "style flex" and manage your behaviors to improve interpersonal relationships. Basic versions of the DISC assessment can be found online.

The MBTI personality inventory was developed in the early 1960s by Isabel Briggs Myers and her mother, Katharine Cook Briggs (1962), building on the work of Carl Jung. "The essence of the theory is that much seemingly random variation in behavior is actually quite orderly and consistent, being due to basic differences in the ways individuals prefer to use their perception and judgment" (Myers & Briggs Foundation, 2019).

The CliftonStrengths (formerly Gallup) Assessment identifies your unique sequence of 34 themes of talent and shows you how to succeed by developing them into CliftonStrengths (Gallup Strengths Center, 2018).

According to Casciaro, Gino, and Kouchaki (2016),

> most people have a dominant motivational focus—what psychologists refer to as either a "promotion" or a "prevention" mindset. Those in the former category think primarily about the growth, advancement, and accomplishments that networking can bring them, while those in the latter see it as something they are obligated to take part in for professional reasons. (p. 105)

Further,

> If you are an introvert, you can't simply will yourself to be extroverted, of course. But everyone can choose which motivational focus to bring to networking. Concentrate on the positives—how it's going to help boost the knowledge and skills that are needed in your job—and the activity will begin to seem much more worthwhile. (p. 105)

SEEKING TO ADVANCE PROFESSIONALLY

If you want to advance beyond a basic nursing role, there are many nursing specialties to consider. With additional training, you can specialize in the area of your interest. As with any higher education or specialty training, you will be required to pass a series of exams and fulfill a period of on-the-job training. Once you decide on a specialization, you'll need to research the requirements. Consider joining a local chapter of the specialty's professional organization to network with those who are already practicing in the area. Through your connection with your local chapter, you will have the opportunity to attend in-person meetings or perhaps be part of an online discussion group that will be relevant to your practice. You can learn much more by networking with colleagues than is possible from a brief description on a website or brochure.

While the importance of networking has been established, literature suggests that networking offers fewer benefits for women. Forret and Dougherty (2004) found that "involvement in networking behavior was more beneficial for the career progress of males than of females" (p. 431). They further note that women build less effective networks than men with less influential and powerful contacts, and they suggest that such ineffectiveness is primarily attributable to women being at a structural disadvantage based on work–family conflict and *homophily*, which is a preference to interact with others whom individuals perceive to be similar to themselves.

Greguletz (Greguletz et al., 2019) argues:

> … a second dimension concerns women's *personal hesitation* to instrumentalize their social ties, eventually resulting in lower levels of network effectivity. Such intrinsic hesitation builds on two main drivers: *relational morality*, denoting women's tendencies to avoid over-benefiting through networking, and *gendered modesty*, denoting how women underestimate their own value in professional contexts. (p. 3)

How can women overcome gender and psychosocial barriers? A qualitative study by Sexton, Lemak, and Wainio (2014) analyzed the career trajectories of successful female healthcare executives to determine factors that generated inflections in their careers. Their findings revealed 25 inflection points, including education and training, experience, career management, family, networking, and mentorship and sponsorship. Most executives mentioned they were involved in professional organizations, at both the national and local levels, during their early and midcareer stages. Women's groups were another area of networking frequently mentioned by the executives. These types of personal networks provided social support and professional development. Their social networks became more strategic and expanded outside the organization as the executives ascended to senior positions.

WAYS TO NETWORK

There are many ways to network, and each has distinct benefits. Time, place, and distance are important factors in selecting which way will work best.

Elevator Speech

An elevator speech can be very beneficial as you build your personal "brand." An elevator speech is a short, clear message about yourself. It communicates who you are and how you contribute to a company or organization. It should be no more than 2 minutes long—imagine yourself running into a potential mentor or employer in an elevator. You need to tell them the essentials about yourself before that ride ends!

It's a good idea to practice your elevator speech aloud, and even to memorize it. Ask a friend to listen and offer suggestions. The more you practice, the more natural you'll sound, and the more comfortable you'll be with seizing the opportunity to present yourself at a moment's notice (University of California, Small Farm Program, n.d.).

The elements of a good elevator speech:

- Begin by clearly articulating your name.
- State your role.
- Briefly describe the company or organization where you work.
- List a few of your accomplishments.

For example:

> I'm Lisa Smith, registered nurse at Children's Hospital, where I've worked for 5 years, providing care for pediatric oncology patients. I've had the pleasure of participating in several initiatives to improve patient outcomes and enhance our patients' hospital experience.

Depending on the occasion, tailor your message to fit the circumstances. At a career fair, you can use your speech to introduce yourself to prospective employers:

> It's nice to meet you. I'm Tiana Mendez. I'm a registered nurse specializing in orthopedic patient care. I'm looking for opportunities to share my expertise and learn new approaches in rehabilitation.

If you're introducing yourself to a patient for the first time:

> Good morning, Mr. Elony. My name is Vihaan Bir. I'm your nurse here at ABC Hospital today. I've taken care of patients on this unit

for 4 years. My colleague, Carol, has given me an update on your progress overnight, and I want to help you achieve your goals for today.

Your message will be different when you meet and introduce yourself to someone new at a conference:

Hello, I'm Susan Ghee. I'm a clinical nurse specialist at XYZ Memorial Hospital in Shah, Georgia, and I'm interested in bringing some new best practices back to my coworkers from this presentation.

Building Collegial Relationships

Often, you network without even consciously thinking about it—for example, when you discuss a topic of interest at your place of employment. Exchanging information with coworkers from different departments or areas of the organization to pursue the topic is an example of networking.

Mary Jo Gumbel, BSN, RN, CPN, a clinical nurse expert, shares a personal story:

"Networking" is a foreign term for a bedside clinical nurse like myself. When I hear this verbiage I envision "businesswomen/ men" gathering over drinks, trading business cards, and discussing clients and quarterly reports. It's hard to envision what networking would look like for someone who wears scrubs and a stethoscope every day while caring for patients and families as their line of work. However, when I truly think about what networking is—sharing common interests, experiences, et cetera—I find that is literally what I do every day as a nurse! When I receive report from the floor nurse about a pre-op patient and develop the safest plan to prep them for surgery—that is networking. When attending shared governance meetings with representatives from every area of the hospital to discuss retention, rewards and recognition, fiscal responsibility—that is networking. One of my favorite times that I really felt like I was networking in the traditional sense was at the ANCC Magnet® Conference in 2018. Our Magnet Program Manager coordinated tabletop discussions between several children's hospitals in the nation to share best practices on various topics, mainly concerning shared governance. It was so eye-opening and exciting to see what others are doing to engage staff, hold everyone accountable, and utilize their leadership to the utmost capacity to strengthen their local shared governance. Networking may be the term commonly used in the business world reserved for happy hours, but in our profession it's ingrained into what we do all day every day. (M. Gumbel, personal communication, August 27, 2019)

In her President's Message titled "Building Relationships: The Power of Networking," Kathleen Carlson, RN, CEN, FAEN (2016) offers,

Whether you are a new graduate, a registered nurse seeking new opportunities, or someone who is just keeping your options open, never underestimate the power of building your professional network! Shared experiences and emotional support can help you realize you are not alone. Make an effort to meet new people and strike up conversations because you never know who will help you in your career down the road or who YOU will be able to help. The opportunities are endless. (p. 295)

SUCCESS STORY

Maureen (Mickey) Mullin, MSN, RN, NEA-BC

Senior Manager, Talent Acquisition, Children's Hospital of Philadelphia, Philadelphia

Maureen (Mickey) Mullin has enjoyed a successful career in oncology and pediatric nursing and has aided nurses in roles as a nursing career specialist. She describes her personal story about networking:

The word "networking" meant nothing to me in my years as a bedside nurse. It was a thing business people did; it wasn't relevant for clinicians. Boy, was I mistaken. Reflecting now as a seasoned nurse and manager in Human Resources, I was networking all along the way but didn't recognize it. It started in my clinical rotations in nursing school. I connected with the nurses and the manager on a very desirable unit—it was difficult to land a position as a new graduate on this unit but somehow I did and firmly believe the connections on the rotation helped. I was thrilled to work with such amazing nurses on a unit with a great reputation. My preceptor was phenomenal and helped me form an outstanding clinical foundation and set the expectations for future patient care experiences.

I strived to be the best nurse possible and was recognized with a hospital award during Nurses Week. That recognition resulted in a connection with the Director of Nursing (in those days this was the highest ranking nurse, and equivalent to the Chief Nursing Officer we see today). Based on her recognizing my award and effort, she later reached out to me after moving to a new hospital and offered me a promotion. I was thrilled and followed her and the opportunity trail. Although it didn't work out as expected, the experience was worthwhile and the lesson of connections was beginning to emerge. But I still didn't see it as the unfamiliar "networking."

Mickey continues,

In my next position as a staff nurse on a surgical unit, we received many transfers from ICU. The ICU nurses were recognized for their expertise with our sickest patients. I respected and admired them but never saw myself as one of them. I asked questions and learned what I could from them to help our patients, developing friendly relationships along the way. Based on these frequent handoffs and increasing familiarity, one particularly supportive ICU nurse suggested a transfer to ICU. I was stunned—and scared to death—but she promised the team would support and teach me. That connection was all I needed to take the next step and move out of my comfort zone. They were amazing and taught me many lessons, beginning with stepping out of your comfort zone.

When I later became involved in committees, which eventually turned into Shared Governance, the connections with nurses from other units and leaders just developed as part of the work. This is where clinical nurses can practice their networking skills, connecting through the team work and building relationships. I volunteered often and never said no when asked to participate in special projects. Although not purposeful, this further increased my network at work—with an added benefit of many new friends and mentors, too.

Life brought changes, propelling me to make changes in my career. I advanced my education, with subsequent role and responsibility changes. As I progressed through the leadership trajectory, I began to see the value in networking not only at my organization but at school and through professional organizations. I tried to optimize the networking while being careful to never jeopardize my integrity or take advantage of my colleagues. At this point, the *conscious* networking began. The selection of clinical practicums in graduate school presented an opportunity for building a relationship for future opportunities.

As part of my job at the time, I was invited to an event at my graduate school to see the new state-of-the-art simulation lab. I should mention, I was tired and didn't really feel like attending on that cold, rainy night after working all day, but I pushed myself because you never know what might come of it. I was very interested in teaching online at this school and wondered if I would see anyone, so I threw a resume in my bag just in case. I noticed one of my online professors and introduced myself. We shared a wonderful conversation and when I mentioned my future interest, she suggested I work with the Dean of Nursing.

The dean at the time was Gloria Donnelly, a well-known, brilliant and innovative leader in nursing education whom I had met at several professional meetings but did not have any relationship with. The thought of working with her completely intimidated me but my professor pushed the idea, and me. The professor reintroduced me to Dean Donnelly and I later emailed my request to meet and discuss the possibilities. Unbelievably, she accepted my request to meet and offered to serve as my preceptor. Wow! Just like moving to ICU, I was again really pushing myself. The dean pushed me too, but she was supportive and challenging at the same time. It was an extraordinary experience and my goal to teach online was realized, but the real outcome was an ongoing mentor relationship with an improbable friend which started when a goal met an opportunity through networking.

After 27 years at the same institution and lots of organizational changes, it was time to move on, but at this point I was entrenched in best practice and the Magnet® philosophy and only wanted to consider the best places to work. At a regional meeting of my professional organization, I mentioned my intentions to a few selected colleagues from exceptional organizations. Two suggested I send a resume and queried me on what I was really interested in doing. As we moved through the process, I was eventually hired for a role I would never have applied to, and it proved the greatest challenge of my career. Again, the networking and moving beyond my comfort zone were critical to my success.

Everyone has a different recipe for success and professional satisfaction. For me it is all about honesty, effort, and relationships. It hasn't failed me yet. (Mullin, M., personal communication, August 18, 2019)

You may need to reach beyond your local peers to explore best practices nationally. If a formal venue doesn't already exist, you can create one! With skill, drive, and determination, you can bring knowledgeable resources together and advance innovative strategies to meet healthcare needs.

SUCCESS STORY

Kellyanne LaFrado, MSN, RN, CPN

Orientation Coordinator & Education Nurse Specialist, Children's Hospital of Philadelphia, Philadelphia, PA

Kellyanne LaFrado describes how her desire to benchmark with other organizations was achieved by networking:

Working in a large metropolitan pediatric hospital as a member of the centralized nursing workforce and caring for patient assignments across the organization, confidence in my communication skills had always been a must. It was essential to be able to meet nurses and identify, in a few minutes, who had the experience to be a resource, who had the brain to help with the technology and who would be willing to sit and discuss at lunch time. The day my colleague approached me for help with a benchmarking project that involved calling organizations to ask some relatively simply questions about workforce orientation I said "yes." Little did I know as a staff nurse then the impact cold calling these pediatric institutions would have in my professional journey.

I started the morning hitting many dead ends as I slowly came to the realization that a centralized work force may be called many different names but mean the same thing. This is a team of nurses and other medical professionals that are assigned based on the needs of the organization to a variety of locations. One particular call I was disconnected three times. I was finally connected with a man who had many letters behind his name. I had no idea what his title or letters really meant. This man suggested I make another call. He indicated that this person was starting to form a collaborative of nurses and, like myself, was interested in sharing best practices. Dolores (Lori) Puttoff called me back and shared with me, not only the orientation answers, but offered to stay in touch and asked if I would join a conference call in the fall with other organizations. I again said "yes."

The call started and I began to discover that teams like mine from across the country had the same struggles and questions we had. After that call, Lori and I spoke by email; she asked if anyone was interested in forming a more formal group. I again said, "Yes." Lori's initial drive and passion was contagious. Initially our group was titled the "Float Pool Collaborative." As we pushed the work forward, I was able to obtain my master's degree and now educated the centralized nurses in my organization. This group has been invaluable in my work as an educator and in orientation of new staff. With Lori and the rest of the team, we have changed our name to the National Collaborative for Healthcare Resource Teams. What started as a call to one individual has connected me to a network of over 150 peers across the nation. What started as a small collaborative is the ground work of what we hope to be a future professional organization to support the best practices of this unique group of nurses and resource staff. (K. LaFrado, personal communication, August 22, 2019)

Attending Social Events

When you hand out a business card at a social event designed to provide opportunities for new collaborations to achieve a mutual goal, you are networking. By sharing your passion, you build relationships with those who are mutually interested in the same issue.

Here's a personal story from Elizabeth Froh, that illustrates the potential of an opportunity when you meet someone who shares your interests.

SUCCESS STORY

Elizabeth Froh, PhD, RN

Nurse Scientist, Center for Pediatric Nursing Research and Evidence-Based Practice, Children's Hospital of Philadelphia, Philadelphia

As a new graduate clinical nurse in the neonatal intensive care unit, I cared for infants with various congenital anomalies. However, it was during the period of time when the infants were ready for enteral feedings that I observed many were fed infant formula and additionally, many were not feeding by mouth but rather by a feeding tube. I had a simple (or so I thought at the time) question: Why? I completed a search of the literature and read numerous articles published by a nurse researcher with the University of Pennsylvania and Children's Hospital of Philadelphia, Dr. Diane Spatz, PhD, RN-BC, FAAN.

I knew immediately that I wanted to talk to Dr. Spatz and her team about my clinical questions. Serendipitously, the university was hosting a graduate open house at the School of Nursing for the doctoral program and Dr. Spatz was one of the faculty that would be presenting during the program. Without hesitation, I registered for the open house and started planning how I could engage Dr. Spatz in conversation. Throughout the program, I kept my head up and saw an opportunity present itself over the lunch hour. Our dialogue was effortless and Dr. Spatz encouraged me to pursue my research interests and to expand my clinical experiences caring for this vulnerable population. So that same afternoon we walked across the street to Children's Hospital of Philadelphia and were welcomed in the office of the nursing leadership of the Newborn/Infant Intensive Care Unit. Although the meeting was brief, the excitement was palpable and I was mentally drafting my applications for both a clinical nursing position on the surgical team at Children's Hospital of Philadelphia and for the 2009 cohort of Penn Nursing's MSN-PhD program.

When anyone asks me how I came to be a Nurse Scientist, I always start with a version of this same story. Mine is a story that highlights how clinical inquiry can be fostered and supported through networking and collaboration. And how that same collaboration can be simultaneously transformed into lasting mentorship. I am forever grateful for the welcome Dr. Spatz gave me, and my questions, that day at the University of Pennsylvania. And I have taken the openness she, and many of my professors, colleagues, peers, family and friends have modeled for me over the years, to heart. Networking is connectedness. And, it is that connectedness, not just in nursing, but across disciplines, that will continue to build the strength of the nursing profession. (E. Froh, personal communication, August 9, 2019)

Joining a Professional Organization

You network when you become involved in the events and projects of a professional organization. There are many nursing organizations. Here are the names and web addresses of several that might interest you:

- American Nurses Association, www.nursingworld.org
- American Association of Colleges of Nursing, www.aacnnursing .org
- Sigma Theta Tau, www.sigmanursing.org
- National League for Nursing, www.nln.org

- International Council of Nurses, www.icn.ch
- Oncology Nursing Society, www.ocn.org
- Emergency Nurses Association, www.ena.org
- Association of Perioperative Registered Nurses, www.aorn.org

Many organizations have local chapters that offer networking and continuing education opportunities. Attending local and regional meetings can be a great way to network in your area and increase your knowledge. Some organizations offer financial assistance to attend conferences and seminars.

Here's my personal story: When I began my nursing career at a National Cancer Institute (NCI)–designated comprehensive cancer center, I joined the Oncology Nurses Society—both the local chapter and the national organization. The local chapter offered dinner meetings with education programs. I spent time with my coworkers and nurses from local community hospitals that cared for oncology patients. These opportunities to share knowledge helped us all be better oncology nurses. As a member, you can nominate or be nominated to assume an officer role in the leadership of the organization. Doing so can lead to leadership roles at the national level. I met many colleagues who have become a treasured part of my network to this day.

When I became involved in the hospital's journey to Magnet® designation, I joined the American Nurses Association (ANA). The American Nurses Credentialing Center (ANCC), a subsidiary of the ANA, credentials both organizations and individuals who advance nursing. The ANCC administers the Magnet Recognition Program® and designates organizations worldwide where nursing leaders successfully align their nursing strategic goals to improve the organization's patient outcomes.

As a staff nurse, I was asked by Joanne Hambleton, then director of nursing at Fox Chase Cancer Center, to be part of a team of nurses to capture examples for the hospital's Magnet designation application. The ANCC had formalized the Magnet Recognition Program in 1993, and 18 hospitals had earned the designation by 1999. In 2000, Fox Chase Cancer Center became the 19th hospital in the country to achieve Magnet designation and the first specialty hospital to have this prestigious status. We were so excited and proud of this achievement! We had networked with nurses at Magnet-designated organizations as we prepared our application. In this way, we became knowledgeable resources for colleagues in the Philadelphia region who desired to apply for Magnet designation.

In 2008, we participated in an inaugural meeting with nurse leaders from the region to create the Philadelphia Area Magnet Consortium (PAMC). The consortium was composed of nurse leaders from nine hospitals in the region that had achieved Magnet designation, and one of its purposes was to help all maintain ongoing Magnet designation when reapplying every 4 years. The value of this network of nurse leaders who were invested in advancing the profession of nursing has been immeasurable for me personally and for the healthcare organizations in the region. In fact, meeting and working with Rhoda Redulla in this group led to this opportunity to write this chapter in her book! Many more hospitals have earned Magnet designation and sustained it, in part with the help of this collaborative forum. Several of the members, including myself and a dear colleague, Tina Martin, served at various times as recorder, vice president, and president of the PAMC. As Tina notes,

... being a nurse means there is a whole community of nursing colleagues there to support you. Throughout my nursing career, networking has offered me innovative patient care solutions, career advice, and emotional support. As a nurse, you are never alone. Networking with nurses is an invaluable treasure. (C. Martin, personal communication, August 22, 2019)

When involvement grows beyond the local community, you may meet and communicate with new colleagues via conference call, regional or national meetings, or web conferencing. While in the role of Magnet program director at Fox Chase Cancer Center, I sought to collaborate with nurse leaders from other NCI-designated cancer centers about oncology nursing–sensitive clinical indicators in the ambulatory care setting that could be tracked, trended, and benchmarked nationally. The Magnet Recognition Program manual had been revised and included an increased focus on nursing care and patient outcomes beyond the inpatient setting. With support from Anne Jadwin, assistant vice president of nursing, and working from a list provided by Delinda Pendleton, director of Infection Control and Quality Management, I began to reach out to nursing colleagues invested in quality-improvement initiatives at the centers. Since each of the centers was also on the Magnet journey, all were interested in searching and defining measures that highlighted the value of oncology nurses' contributions to positive patient outcomes. The group developed a charter and structure, officers were nominated, and regular conference calls were held. Forming this network eventually led to an institutional review board (IRB)–approved multisite study focused on the incidence of chemotherapy extravasations. Ultimately, a national benchmark was achieved, and the group's study was published. Along the way, we presented at national conferences, and lasting friendships were formed.

Kathryn Roberts, MSN, RN, CNS, CCRN-K, CCNS, FCCM, finds great value in professional organization memberships. She served on the Board of Directors of the American Association of Critical-Care

Nurses (AACN) from 2008 to 2011, the AACN Certification Corporation board from 2010 to 2011, and as president of the organization from 2012 to 2013. Kathryn offers,

> Joining professional organization(s) is an essential part of your professional growth and development. It affords you the opportunity to develop a network, or as I like to think of it, a "community" of nursing colleagues. This community can be local, regional, national or international in scope—and allows you to develop a network of colleagues you can reach out to with clinical/operational questions, mentoring opportunities (as both a mentee and a mentor). Perhaps most important, it exposes you to diverse perspectives. (K. Roberts, personal communication, September 2, 2019)

Social Media

With the proliferation of electronic platforms for communication, social media is now a great way to network instantaneously. By sharing your professional self on sites such as LinkedIn, you can post your résumé, share professional articles, and comment on posts that others have shared. Facebook and Twitter are also frequently searched by prospective employers seeking potential employees. Be sure to keep your information current, and remember that what you post becomes the image viewers have of you.

You can reach many more people through social media. Madeline Bell, president and CEO of CHOP, created her blog, *Heels of Success*:

> ... to provide some guidance to ambitious women about how to elevate themselves in the workplace, ultimately leading to greater representation for women in the C-Suite and on boards. Having begun my career as a night-shift nurse, I hope that the lessons I've learned along the way can help give other women the tools to succeed at the top of their fields. (M. Bell, http://heelsofsuccess .com, 8/19/19)

Since being named CEO of CHOP, Ms. Bell has been sought out by many aspiring leaders and has authored articles on various topics, including challenges, confidence, leadership, professional growth, starting out, women in the workplace, and work–family balance.

Ms. Bell is also the host of *Breaking Through With Madeline Bell*, a podcast that features interviews with CHOP doctors and scientists as well as philanthropists, innovators, and business and civic leaders. She holds a BSc in nursing from Villanova University and an MSc in organizational dynamics from the University of Pennsylvania.

PRACTICAL ADVICE

Jackie Noll, MSN, RN, CEN, senior director at Children's Hospital of Philadelphia, offers this practical advice for all:

Let's face it, nurses often work in high-cost environments within expensive buildings using expensive equipment; however, the most precious resource is truly the people. The key to providing exceptional healthcare involves how we work with the people both at our side and beyond. In the course of your nursing career, you may be in one of three organizational categories of personnel who deliver health care. You may be in a direct care provider position, a middle management role, or lead larger groups of people at a senior/executive level. A critical skill you will need is learning the value of networking across role levels and then creating the opportunities to make the networking happen.

The value of creating relationships both in and outside of nursing fosters unlimited learning along with developing new professional opportunities for your career. As you approach networking, view each person you meet as an opportunity to build your own capabilities as well as to advance work you support. The clinical care nurse has important practical experience to share with a manager or executive leader about what patients and staff need to achieve successful outcomes. Likewise, the executive leader and manager needs the clinical care staff to see the strategy behind decisions and planning. Each organizational role informs the others in order to create the best processes for our patients.

So take the leap and make a networking strategy. Start with self-reflection and think about what you hope to accomplish. Also, address any insecurities or fears you may have in reaching out to others. To minimize any hesitation, remind yourself how seeking to acknowledge others is a real compliment to the person you are approaching. Start practicing with informal approaches like introducing yourself to those around you in an elevator, coffee line, cafeteria, and so on. Say hello, introduce yourself and your role, and learn what others do who work in your organization. You will be surprised at the connections you may already have in your work. In a more structured way, notice who in your organization has talents you would want to add to your skill set. Reach out in person, or in email, and ask them if they would consider a brief coffee chat to introduce yourself and network. Let them know what you admire about them and see if they would be willing to share their experiences. It is important to note that a networking meeting does not always need to be with someone higher in the organization. A senior leader can equally see talent in more junior staff and ask for the same brief meeting. An example is a senior leader who values the expertise of a less senior member of the staff in the world of social media. Reverse mentoring and networking is a powerful way to build relationships and followers.

Never hesitate to think about line-of-sight responsibility in networking when related to a project. As you manage projects, think about who is ultimately responsible for that work. Embrace your leadership courage and invite the key stakeholder(s) to attend a meeting, review a project plan, or round with you and staff involved in this work. Agosto, Bernstein, Gebeline-Myers, Noll, and Steck (2019) describe how inviting the senior vice presidents to a Shared Governance meeting connected the executives to the frontline staff on managing a goal of financial stewardship. A member of the project team purposely networked and shared the vision with three executive leaders and invited them to offer a 60-second elevator speech to nursing staff who were managing a project. The Chief Nursing Officer, Vice President of Supply Chain, and the Chief Financial Officer all accepted. The ability to network across organizational layers brought two groups together who had the same mission but often were not in the same room together (Agosto et al., 2019). Make networking both informally and formally part of your strategy planning for personal growth and professional matters. (J. Noll, personal communication, September 3, 2019)

CONCLUSION

As with anything of value, maintaining your network takes time, care, and effort. You may see some of your contacts often, especially if they work in your organization. Others may be simply an email or phone call away. You may connect with some annually at a professional conference or seminar. As you become aware of your contacts' interests or special concerns, reach out periodically to show your interest and willingness to be supportive. Keep your network alive by nurturing your relationships.

Ultimately, networking effectively offers mutual benefits to you and those you meet. You can learn a great deal from others, and they can likewise learn from you. Networking helps advance the profession of nursing, and that translates into positive outcomes for nurses and others who want to improve care for patients, their loved ones, and the community.

Key Points

- Effective networking is a powerful tool in advancing your nursing career.
- Be prepared with your elevator speech.
- Create a meaningful network through your professional organizations, social media, or your regular job.

References

Agosto, P., Bernstein, M., Gebeline-Myers, C., Noll, J., & Steck, J. (2019). *Nursing-led savings*. Indianapolis, IN: Sigma Theta Tau International.

Cardillo, D. (n.d.). *How networking can work for you*. Retrieved from https://donnacardillo.com/articles/networkingwork4u/

Carlson, K. (2016). Building relationships: The power of networking. *Journal of Emergency Nursing, 42*(4), 295. doi:10.1016/j.jen.2016.05.005

Casciaro, T., Gino, F., & Kouchaki, M. (2016). Managing yourself: Learn to love networking. *Harvard Business Review, 94*(5), 104–107.

Drake, K. (2017). The power of networking. *Nursing Management, 48*(9), 56. doi:10.1097/01.NJMA.0000522184.39403.65

Forret, M. L., & Dougherty, T. W. (2004). Networking behaviors and career outcomes: Differences for men and women? *Journal of Organizational Behavior, 25*(3), 419–437. doi:10.1002/job.253

Gallup Strengths Center. (2018). *CliftonStrengths*. Retrieved from https://www.gallupstrengthscenter.com/

Greguletz, E., Diehl, M.-R., & Kreutzer, K. (2019). Why women build less effective networks than men: The role of structural exclusion and personal hesitation. *Human Relations, 72*(7), 1234–1261. doi:10.1177/0018726718804303

Marston, W. M. (1928). *Emotions of normal people*. New York, NY: Harcourt, Brace and Co.

Myers, I. B. (1962). *The Myers-Briggs type indicator*. Palo Alto, CA: Consulting Psychologists Press.

The Myers & Briggs Foundation. (2019). *MBTI® basics*. Retrieved from https://www.myersbriggs.org/my-mbti-personality-type/mbti-basics/home.htm?bhcp=1

Sexton, D. W., Lemak, C. H., & Wainio, J. A. (2014). Career inflection points of women who successfully achieved the hospital CEO position. *Journal of Healthcare Management, 59*(5), 367–374. doi:10.1097/00115514-201409000-000111

University of California, Small Farm Program. (n.d.). *The 30 second elevator speech*. Retrieved from http://sfp.ucdavis.edu/files/163926.pdf

11

Self-Care for Nurses

Rhoda R. Redulla and Georgia Giannopoulos

"You cannot keep giving to others if you do not give to yourself, first."
—Leslie K. Lobell

Are you a healthy nurse? A sleepy nurse? A tired nurse? In 2017, the American Nurses Association (ANA) launched the Healthy Nurse, Healthy Nation™ (HNHN) Grand Challenge. HNHN is a social movement designed to transform the health of the nation by improving the health of the nation's 4 million RNs, comprising the majority of healthcare professionals in the hospital setting and providers of the nation's short- and long-term patient care (Raney & Van Zanten, 2019). The program is focused on helping nurses achieve healthy levels of activity, sleep, nutrition, quality of life, and safety. For nurses, this is sometimes challenging to do consistently. Not being at the best state of health can take you away from reaching your full potential as a professional. In this chapter, you will learn about the importance of self-care and advice on how to do it.

SELF-CARE FOR NURSES

Self-care consists of any activity that we do deliberately in order to promote and maintain our mental, emotional, and physical health (Michael, 2018). The ANA Code of Ethics encompasses self-care (Purdue University Global, n.d.). Provision 5 states, "The nurse owes the same duties to self as to others, including the responsibility to promote health and safety, preserve wholeness of character and integrity, maintain competence, and continue personal and professional growth." This inclusion in the Code of Ethics implies the moral duty for nurses to practice self-care. When you skip a lunch break or work extended hours on back-to-back days, you hear others remind you to "take care of yourself." What can you do to take care of yourself? Later in this chapter, you will learn more about specific strategies that you can do and hopefully sustain.

SELF-CARE FOR NURSES: WHY DOES IT MATTER?

Nurses are constantly exposed to stress that can have detrimental effects on their health. Time constraints, heavy workload, multiple tasks and roles, and emotionally challenging moments are just some of the stressors for healthcare workers, including nurses (Ripstein-Leuenberger, Mauthner, Bryan Sexton, & Schwendimann, 2017). The increasing complexity and intensity of nurses' workload makes it even more imperative to advise self-care. Iacono (2010) shared how perianesthesia nurses can have moments, and sometimes hours, of tension and heightened emotion. The pace of their work is dynamic, often unpredictable, and frequently stressful. The healthcare environment is uncertain, with shrinking resources and increased work pressures. Nurses are exposed to patients experiencing pain, suffering, and trauma. Recurrent stress in caregiving professions can lead to compassion fatigue and burnout (Hooper, Craig, Janvrin, Wetsel, & Reimels, 2010). This can impact their health and ability to provide the best possible care. In fact, there is a relationship between nurses' ability to care for self and their ability to provide effective patient care (Iacono, 2010). Evidence has shown that nurses who do participate in self-care activities are more likely to discuss the benefits of being healthy, making healthy choices, and lifestyle changes with their patients, and their patients are more likely to take them seriously (Kahn, 2015).

A national study looked into nurses' physical and mental health, the relationship between health and medical errors, and the association between nurses' perceptions of wellness support and their health. A 53-item survey was disseminated by 10 professional nursing organizations, which sent the information to their members in their electronic newsletter communications. A group of 20 chief nursing officers from large and small hospitals across the United States also distributed information about the survey to their nurses. Over half of the nurses in the study reported suboptimal physical and mental health. Approximately half of the nurses reported having made medical errors in the past 5 years. Compared with nurses with better health, those with worse health were associated with 26% to 71%

higher likelihood of medical errors (Melnyk et al., 2017). The sample size of 1,790 was small relative to the population of nurses in the nation; however, the findings of the study provide important information on the wellness status of nurses and a prompt to explore the link between caregiver wellness and medical errors.

NURSES AS ROLE MODELS OF SELF-CARE

When nurses engage in self-care, they are better able to handle daily stress, practice compassion, improve patient care (Sevier & Randle, 2019), and become great role models to patients and families as we often hear and say, "Practice what you preach." Oncology nurses are spearheading some of the best research and clinical studies on chronic illness and initiatives that help improve patient survival through self-care behaviors (Smith, 2018). However, we are less likely to incorporate these health strategies into our own daily lives (Blum, 2014). Nurses must start to prioritize the care of themselves.

STRATEGIES FOR SELF-CARE

Davis (2018) recommends 12 things to take better care for yourself. I selected some of these tips to highlight here.

1. Make sleep part of your self-care routine. Nurses can have irregular sleep patterns related to being on call and working nights, rotating, or extended shifts. Working night shifts makes nurses vulnerable to negative effects such as insomnia, decreased alertness, cognitive decrement, fatigue, mood disturbance, reproductive issues, increase in accidents, and family, social, and emotional problems (Akerstedt, 1990). While it can be challenging for all of us nurses, we are called to commit to these healthy sleep habits (Larson, 2019).

- Establish a consistent routine. While it is tough with rotating shifts, decide what time you will go to bed each day and what time you plan to wake up. Refrain from deviating from your schedule.
- Ask people not to disturb you. Communicate your expectations to family or household members.
- Make your bedroom sleep-friendly. Keep the room dark and cool when you need to sleep. You can use a white noise or sound machine to help you stay asleep. This may be more helpful for nurses who sleep during the day.
- Forego the electronics before bed. Experts recommend reducing or turning off electronics at least an hour prior to bedtime.

- Be mindful of your caffeine intake. The amount and timing of caffeine you consume can impact how easy it is for you to fall asleep and may also affect your sleep quality. Caffeine is found in beverages such as coffee, tea, cola, energy drinks, and some foods such as chocolate and coffee- or chocolate-flavored ice creams.

- If you drink alcohol, do so in moderation and avoid alcohol for 1 to 2 hours before bed. Remember to stay well hydrated throughout the day by sipping on plain or infused water, too.

- Nap strategically. A 20- to 30-minute nap before work may help you fight sleepiness during your shift.

2. Exercise daily as part of your self-care routine. Choose an activity that you enjoy, whether it's biking, dancing, or brisk walking. With walking, you might be thinking nurses are already putting in a lot of steps at work. You should be doing something in addition to what you do at work. If possible, walk outdoors. Many people need at least 150 minutes per week of moderate-to-vigorous physical activity.

3. Eat right for self-care. Choose nutritious and delicious foods that nourish you and satisfy your taste buds. Aim for balanced meals or snacks that include fruits and vegetables; a protein such as fish, chickpeas, or lentils; whole grains such as brown rice, barley, or quinoa; and healthy fat such as olive oil. Consider bringing pre-portioned snacks to work that include protein, dietary fiber, and healthy fats, such as unsalted nuts—the mix of nutrients will help you sustain your energy levels throughout your shift. Create a healthy food environment at home, and take time to enjoy your meals. If you're looking for some recipe inspiration, check out http://www.nyp.org/nutrition/recipes. In one study of more than 300 nurses by Ross, Bevans, Brooks, Gibbons, and Wallen (2018), results showed that almost half of the nurses' self-report could be characterized as not eating a healthy diet.

4. Say no to others, and say yes to your self-care. Many of us can struggle to say no. The next time you are torn and tempted to say yes to something that is unnecessary, think of the time when you had too much on your plate and you felt overwhelmed.

5. Take a self-care trip. One of the best tips I have received for self-care is to visit a place you have not seen before at least once a year. Take that a step further and plan to go on a trip to unwind and rejuvenate as often as you can.

6. Let a pet help you with your self-care. Having a pet can reduce stress and help you relax. Dogs can decrease feelings of anxiety and even blood pressure. Animal-assisted therapy (AAT) has been used in various settings. With AAT, patients have achieved positive outcomes such as feeling happy, feeling relaxed, and feeling calm (Brown et al., 2019). In one randomized controlled

trial (RCT), dogs, cats, dolphins, birds, cows, rabbits, ferrets, and guinea pigs were used in AAT (Kamioka et al., 2014).

7. Take care of yourself by getting organized. This entails planning and preparing your meals and organizing your home so you don't spend time on other things that will take you away from your self-care activity.

OTHER SELF-CARE PRACTICES

Resilience

Three Good Things exercise is a resilience-building intervention that involves asking the questions "What are three things that went well today?" and "What was your role in bringing them about?" Several studies have been conducted among nurses, physicians, and other healthcare professionals implementing this exercise. Study participants were asked to respond to these questions for 14 days through an online survey. In one study involving neonatal intensive care unit (NICU) healthcare professionals (including nurses), three main themes were identified from the responses: (a) having a good day at work, (b) having supportive relationships, and (c) having meaningful use of self-determined time. The Three Good Things exercise acknowledges the importance of self-care in healthcare, can promote well-being, and might ultimately enhance resilience (Rippstein-Leeuenberger, Mauthner, Sexton, & Schwendimann, 2017).

Mindfulness

In *A Book That Takes Its Time: An Unhurried Adventure to Mindfulness*, the authors invite readers to take time to read, take time to create, take time to reflect, and take time to let go. These are just a few proposals on ways you can "take time" (Smit & Van der Hulst, 2017).

The use of mindfulness-based stress reduction (MBSR) may be a key intervention to help improve nurses' ability to cope with stress and ultimately improve the quality of patient care provided. In a review of the literature by Smith (2014), empirical evidence regarding utilizing MBSR with nurses and other healthcare professionals suggests several positive benefits, including decreased stress, burnout, and anxiety and increased empathy, focus, and mood. Mindfulness interventions included:

Body Scan: Monitoring of the body to increase awareness of sensations ("being aware of your body's present state of being")

How this is done: You can do this while sitting, lying down, or in other postures. Research recommends that you need 20 to 45 minutes to do this three or four times a week for the best benefit

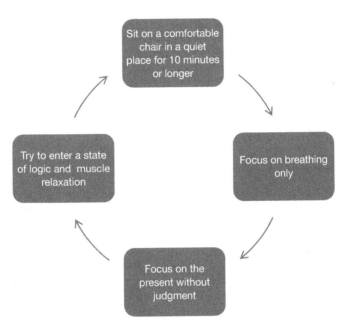

Figure 11.1 Mindfulness sitting meditation

(Greater Good Science Center, 2017). However, when you are crunched for time, there are 3- or 5-minute versions of the body scan. For an example of a script for a body scan, visit the UCLA Mindful Awareness Research Center website (https://www .uclahealth.org/marc/mindful-meditations).

Mindfulness Sitting Meditation (MSM): Mindful attention to breathing with nonjudgmental awareness of thoughts and distractions in the mind. MSM focuses on the physical sensation of breathing, and sitting meditation is a common technique and easy to experience for those who are new to it (Figure 11.1). It differs from meditation in other physical movement forms, such as tai chi, qigong, yoga, or mindful walking (Liu, Qui, & Louie, 2017).

How it is done:
— May or may not incorporate music
— May or may not close eyes
— May or may not sit in Zen position
— May practice daily at your own pace

Hatha Yoga: It is a type of yoga that comes to mind when you think of "yoga" in general terms. It is most appropriate for those who have never been trained to do yoga (Chanta, Klaewsongcram, Mickleborough, & Tongtako, 2019). Hatha yoga is the physical training portion, combined with postural exercise, deep breathing and relaxation, and meditation.

Mindfulness involves intentional activation of loving-kindness, gratitude, and self-compassion (Halm, 2017). The studies showed overall improvement in physiological and psychological well-being. Physiologically, nurses reported increased relaxation states and fewer physical symptoms after MBSR programs.

THE NURSE LEADER'S ROLE IN SELF-CARE

If not yet obvious, the role of the nurse leader in self-care is to be a role model and facilitator for the team. I am fortunate to experience this firsthand through my manager, Beverly Karas-Irwin, DNP, RN, NP-C, HNB-BC, NEA-BC, director of nursing excellence. Beverly starts every meeting with an invitation to take a deep, cleansing breath. For longer meetings or retreats, she asks one of us in the group to prepare and lead the intention. After a few meetings doing this, I have started to look forward to this time with the team. Our team is composed of Magnet® program directors. To say at the very least, we work under tight timelines and things can be quite intense. I appreciate how my manager commits to leading the team in this quick, simple self-care activity.

Another nurse leader colleague, Peter Stoffan, MPA, BSN, RN, CCRN, NEA-BC, patient care director, has championed self-care within his team and across the organization. Peter was featured on the Healthy Nurse Healthy Nation newsletter, where he shared his commitment to creating and maintaining a healthy work environment. In 2017, Peter launched a "Holiday Health Reset" for a full week after Thanksgiving and made this as a tradition for his team moving forward (Carpenter, 2019). Here is a sample menu of activities:

- On "Meditation Monday," staff were led in meditation via apps with various aromatherapies. This was a staff favorite and will remain so. It's always a good way to start the week off!
- Tuesday had a healthy-eating focus, where staff learned about the spice turmeric and shared their favorite turmeric recipes. The year 2018 included a kombucha-making class.
- Wednesday Peter invited our NYP*BeHealthy* (an internal wellness program) well-being coaches up to the unit to measure employees' body mass index (BMI) and waist circumference and provide one-on-one well-being coaching. This visit on the unit made it convenient for staff to easily set time aside and cover each other for the 1:1 counseling. Ongoing 1:1 coaching sessions continue.

- Thursday was "Pilates With Peter." As a licensed Pilates instructor, Peter led the staff in basic and convenient Pilates moves and taught about good spine health.
- Friday ended the week with the healing power of music, as Peter partnered with the hospital "Music and Medicine" group to give a concert to staff.

WORKPLACE CAMPAIGNS

In one study, the impact of self-monitoring and a poster campaign was examined. Twenty-six hospital nurses from four different hospital units were provided a digital step counter, a handout that listed the physical activity guidelines, and a personal activity report. Healthy lifestyle promotions such as encouraging use of the stairs instead of the elevator, tips for increasing fiber consumption, and active break instructional exercise posters were used to guide and motivate the nurse participants. Baseline testing was completed prior to and post intervention, which included a Situational Motivational Scale (SIMS) and International Physical Activity Questionnaire. SIMS was used to measure participants' intrinsic motivation, internal regulation, external regulation, and amotivation (no intention to be physically active). In addition, weight, blood pressure, resting heart rate, and waist and hip circumference measurements were also obtained pre- and postintervention. Study results showed that participants' moderate to vigorous physical activity and step count increased (Raney & Van Zanten, 2019).

SUCCESS STORY

Stephanie Nolan, DNP, MBA, RN, CPAN, NEA-BC

I am incredibly fortunate and grateful for all the roads that have led me to today.

Unbeknown to my younger self, my journey through nursing was not planned and sometimes quite unexpected. My nursing background is critical care, both adults and pediatrics. I spent most of my years as a postanesthesia care unit (PACU) nurse and spent over 10 years volunteering as a PACU nurse on various medical missions all over the world. My original "plan" was to go back to graduate school and become a certified registered nurse anesthetist (CRNA), yet over time I was approached to take on various forms of leadership roles. What I didn't expect was that I truly enjoyed leadership and being able to make a positive change in nursing, so I happily embraced more opportunities when they arose.

Charge nurse led to chairing committees, which eventually led to clinical nurse manager, nurse manager, and now director of nursing. The joy from watching a team bring their best every day to provide exceptional, high-quality care to patients, while continuing to find ways to advance the nursing profession, is beyond extraordinary.

Why do you invest in self-care?

As nurses, caring for ourselves is vital to bringing our best every day. Our jobs as nurses is to promote better health for patients. We absolutely need to do the same for ourselves. For me, starting out the day on a positive note is important. The first thing I do to start my day is write a note of gratitude in my journal, which sets the tone for my day. Exercise has always been a large part of my life, as I grew up playing sports. As I got older, exercise remained a large part of my life but for very different reasons. I have always loved to run. Running for me now is more about mental health and mindfulness than it is about the physical competition. I run early in the morning to start my day and disconnect. Living in New York City, I've few quiet, mindful moments. Being able to start my day watching the sunrise over a quiet NYC brings me incredible peace and joy. I try never to take that moment for granted, no matter what is going on in my life at the time.

Additionally, I like to challenge myself and push myself outside of my comfort zone at least one time a year. Whether it's a race I have never run, a triathlon, or a dance class I want to try, I commit to one new thing every year. Right now I am committed to mastering the crow pose in yoga! Pushing myself out of my comfort zone builds my self-confidence, which in turn builds self-esteem and dissipates any negative self-talk. Quite frankly, mastering the crow prose for me is a long shot, and whether I ever do it correctly isn't really what matters to me. I am proud of myself for continuing to try every class.

Self-care is not only about exercise for me; it's about nutrition but also rest. I am a classic overcommitter and have learned to say "no" more and without guilt. It's about listening to not only your body but your mind that's typically giving a signal that it's time to slow down and recharge.

Self-care is a journey. I grew into these habits with periods of time that I admittedly was not caring for myself well and had some unhealthy habits and behaviors. What I learned is that self-care is incredibly important, and with anything it's about progress, not perfection. What works for me may not work for you. How you choose to care for yourself is up to you and only you. I can say assuredly you will never regret investing in yourself.

What is your advice for nurses?

My advice to nurses is to be open to all possibilities. Anything is possible. Volunteer to take on roles. Do something out of your comfort zone. Be very open and receptive to honest feedback, both giving and receiving, as that is how you learn and grow.

Nursing is a team sport; no one nurse can carry it all. Be a team player and be kind to everyone, including all the support services you work with every day. Nurses would not be successful without all of our support services assisting us each and every day.

Be inclusive and embrace the differences. Everyone has strengths. Diverse thinking is what stimulates innovation. Oftentimes the best idea comes from the unlikeliest source.

Join your professional organization and network. You would be surprised how we all struggle with similar challenges but also how willing nurses are to share best practices and help each other when they can. Nurses working together is how we will continue to advance the nursing profession.

Lastly, invest in yourself, continue to learn, and do what makes your heart happy.

Doctoral work on healthy nurse leaders

When I started the DNP program, I knew I wanted to research some aspect of health behaviors of nurses and nurse leaders. The American Nurses Association (ANA) Enterprise had previously published results concerning health behaviors and threats to nurses' health. For my scholarly project, I was incredibly fortunate to partner with the ANA and their Healthy Nurse, Healthy Nation™ initiative. Together, we researched the health behaviors of nurse leaders, as leaders in nursing are essentially responsible for creating the healthy work environments that set the team up for success. The results can be found in ANA's *American Nurse Today*, January 2020, in an article titled "The HealthyNurse® Leader: How Do the Health Behaviors of Nurse Leaders Measure Up?"

References

Akerstedt T. (1990). Psychological and psychophysiological effects of shift work. *Scandinavian Journal of Work, Environment and Health, 16*(Suppl. 1), 67–73. doi:10.5271/sjweh.1819

American Nurses Association. (2015). *Code of ethics for nurses with interpretive statements.* Silver Spring, MD: Author.

Blum, C. (2014). Practicing self-care for nurses: A nursing program initiative. *The Online Journal of Issues in Nursing.* Retrieved from http://ojin.nursingworld.org/MainMenuCategories/ANAMarketplace/ANAPeriodicals/OJIN/TableofContents/Vol-19-2014/No3-Sept-2014/Practicing-Self-Care-for-Nurses.html

Brown, S., Snelders, J., Godbold, J., Moran-Peters, J., Driscoll, D., Donoghue, D., . . . Eckardt, S. (2019). Effects of animal-assisted activity on mood states and feelings in a psychiatric setting. *Journal of the American Psychiatric Nurses Association*, 1078390319853617. doi:10.1177/1078390319853617

Carpenter, H. (2019). *Healthy nurse spotlight: Peter Stoffan.* Retrieved from https://engage.healthynursehealthynation.org/blogs/13/3063

Chanta, A., Klaewsongcram, J., Mickleborough, T., & Tongtako, W. (2019). Effect of Hatha yoga training on rhinitis symptoms and cytokines in allergic rhinitis patients. *Asian Pacific Journal of Allergy and Immunology.* doi:10.12932/AP-260419-0547

Davis, T. (2018). *Self-care: 12 ways to take better care of yourself.* Retrieved from https://www.psychologytoday.com/us/blog/click-here-happiness/201812/self-care-12-ways-take-better-care-yourself

Greater Good Science Center. (2017). *A 3-minute body scan meditation to cultivate mindfulness.* Retrieved from https://www.mindful.org/a-3-minute-body-scan-meditation-to-cultivate-mindfulness/

Halm, M. (2017). The role of mindfulness in enhancing self-care for nurses. *American Journal of Critical Care, 26*(4), 344–348. doi:10.4037/ajcc2017589

Hooper, C., Craig, J., Janvrin, D. R., Wetsel, M. A., & Reimels, E. (2010). Compassion satisfaction, burnout, and compassion fatigue among emergency nurses compared with nurses in other selected inpatient specialties. *Journal of Emergency Nursing, 36*(5), 420–427. doi:10.1016/j.jen.2009.11.027

Iacono, M. (2010). Nurses' self-care: A question of balance. *American Society of Perianesthesia Nurses, 25*(3), 174–176. doi:10.1016/j.jopan.2010.03.007

Kahn, S. (2015). Healthy nurse healthy nation. *Visionary Leadership* [Video file]. Retrieved from https://vimeo.com/149328192

Kamioka, H., Okada, S., Tsutani, K., Park, H., Okuizumi, H., Handa, S., . . . Mutoh, Y. (2014). Effectiveness of animal-assisted therapy: A systematic review of randomized controlled trials. *Complementary Therapies in Medicine, 22*(2), 371–390. doi:10.1016/j.ctim.2013.12.016

Larson, J. (2019). *How to sleep better: 10 tips for nurses.* Retrieved from https://www.travelnursing.com/news/features-and-profiles/how-to-sleep-better-10-tips-for-nurses/

Liu, S., Qiu, G., & Louie, W. (2017). Use of mindfulness sitting meditation in Chinese American Women in treatment of cancer. *Integrative Cancer Therapy, 16*(1), 110–117. doi:10.1177/1534735416649661

Melnyk, B. M., Orsolini, L., Tan, A., Arslanian-Engoren, C., Melkus, G. D., Dunbar-Jacob, J., . . . Lewis, L. M. (2018). A national study links nurses' physical and mental health to medical errors and perceived worksite wellness. *Journal of Occupational and Environmental Medicine, 60*(2), 126–131. doi:10.1097/JOM.0000000000001198

Michael, R. (2018). *What self-care is—And what it isn't.* Retrieved from https://psychcentral.com/blog/what-self-care-is-and-what-it-isnt-2/

Purdue University Global. (n.d.). *The importance of self-care for nurses and how to put a plan in place.* Retrieved from https://www.purdueglobal.edu/blog/nursing/self-care-for-nurses/

Raney, M., & Van Zanten, E. (2019). Self-care posters serve as a low-cost option for physical activity promotion of hospital nurses. *Society for Public Health Education, 20*(3), 354–362. doi:10.1177/1524839918763585

Ripstein-Leuenberger, K., Mauthner, O., Bryan Sexton, J., & Schwendimann, R. (2017). A qualitative analysis of three good things intervention in healthcare workers. *BMJ Open, 7*(5), e015826. doi:10.1136/bmjopen-2017-015826

Ross, A., Bevans, M., Brooks, A., Gibbons, S., & Wallen, G. (2018). Nurses and health-promoting behaviors: Knowledge may not translate into self-care. *AORN Journal, 105*(3), 267–275. doi:10.1016/j.aorn.2016.12.018

Sevier, C., & Randle, V. (2019). The importance of self-care. *Georgia Nursing.* Retrieved from https://www.nursingald.com/publications/1869

Smit, I., & Van der Hulst, A. (2017). *A book that takes its time.* Sanoma Media Netherlands.

Smith, M. (2018). Practice what you preach: Nurses' self-care. *Oncology Nursing News.* Retrieved from https://www.oncnursingnews.com/contributor/maggie-smith/2018/12/practice-what-you-preach-nurses-self-care

Smith, S. A. (2014). Mindfulness-based stress reduction: An intervention to enhance the effectiveness of nurses' coping with work-related stress. *International Journal of Nursing Knowledge, 25*(2), 119–130. doi:10.1111/2047-3095.12025

12

Career Opportunities for Nurses

Avis M. Russ

"From Patient Care Director, I became a Director of Nursing; and from Director of Nursing, I became VP of Patient Services and CNO. I look forward to learning, leading and serving in this essential healthcare executive role; and I am resolute and excited that the end of my career remains unwritten."

—Ophelia Byers, DNP, RN, WHNP-BC, RNC-OB, NEA-BC

Taking advantage of opportunities, whether in nursing or outside of nursing, is not just about finding a job but about building and managing a career that will span three to five decades. To say that managing a career takes time and effort is an understatement. This chapter provides information and guidance for managing a planned, and sometimes unplanned, career path in nursing and capitalizing on opportunities that are available to today's nurses. Career "opportunity" includes any action that promotes self-actualization, advances your career, or enhances your earning potential, whether the opportunity is in your current position or in an advanced role.

NURSING AS A CAREER: THE PROGRESSION OF NURSING AS A PROFESSION

According to the Bureau of Labor Statistics, approximately 3 million RNs were employed in the United States in 2016. Between 2016 and 2026, the projected job growth for RNs is 15%. This increase is due to an aging population in the United States and the prevalence of health conditions related to aging (Bureau of Labor Statistics, n.d.). A well-prepared and experienced nursing workforce will be there to meet this challenge, and the opportunities that will be created as a result are many. Being well prepared means taking deliberate steps toward professional development. The American Nurses Credentialing Center's (ANCC) Magnet Model' Structural Empowerment Domain articulates the RN's role as a lifelong learner, including the pursuit of certifications in one's specialty and advanced degrees, impacting positive changes in nursing practice through nurses' affiliations with professional organizations, and active participation in decision-making groups (ANCC, 2017).

In the not-too-distant past, nursing was viewed as one of the few viable career options for women—along with teaching and clerical roles. Characteristically viewed in the past as a doctors' helper role, nursing has become a highly skilled profession for both women and men, guided by evidence-based standards of practice and autonomous decision-making. Nursing has always been highly regarded by the public as a noble profession, propelled by organizations such as Gallup through its survey initiatives. Results of occupation-focused Gallup surveys have elevated public awareness of nursing as a respected career. The most recent Gallup survey results on honesty and ethics conducted in December 2018 showed that "more than four in five Americans (84%) rated the honesty and ethical standards of nurses as 'very high' or 'high'" (Brenan, 2019). Nursing was at the top of the list of 20 professions. The second highest percentage was for medical doctors at 67%. The 2018 survey was the 17th consecutive year that nurses were rated highest.

It is no surprise that nursing as a career choice has been on the upswing since the early 2000s due to: (a) the high regard for nursing by the public and (b) initiatives such as the 2002 Johnson & Johnson Campaign for Nursing's Future. This initiative put a spotlight on nurses and their contributions to healthcare.[4] In the past decade, millennials as a group were drawn to nursing as a career, influenced in part by economic events such as the 2008 recession and the positive publicity that nursing has received. The benefits of nursing as a career include the fact that the profession provides for a stable income, job security, an ever-expanding number of settings to practice, and a wide variety of positions in hospitals. Despite these factors, nursing has also had its share of shortages that seem to be cyclical. The next predicted cycle is an imminent one created by the number of baby boomer nurses (those born between 1946 and 1964) who will retire in the next decade or two. The good news is some nurses who are of retirement age and *can* retire will remain in the workforce on a part-time or per diem basis. Because there are numerous roles and opportunities that nurses can pursue both inside and outside of hospitals, nurses may be more likely to remain in the workforce, albeit in different roles than they occupied in their preretirement years.

WHERE NURSES WORK AND NURSES' COMPENSATION

Hospitals remain the number one workplace for nurses, but opportunities exist in a variety of settings, including physicians' offices, home healthcare services, skilled nursing facilities, and outpatient care facilities. In May 2018 the median annual wage for RNs was $71,730, and the top five industries where nurses were employed are listed in Table 12.1 (Brenan, 2019; Bureau of Labor Statistics, n.d.).

The American Nurses Association's report titled "Nursing by the Numbers" states that nurses work in approximately 137 industries, with the vast majority working in hospitals (McMenamin, 2016). Salaries for nurses have increased exponentially in the last two decades and vary by role, education, and setting. A recent article at the nurse.org website (nurse.org, 2020) lists the 15 top paying nursing jobs (see Box 12.1).

The list does not include nurse executive, nurse leader, or nurse manager positions where salaries are generally in the top salary tiers. In addition to hospital-based direct care nursing positions, there are career opportunities available to nurses that are not as common. For example, nurses can assume roles in forensics, as legal nurse consultants, in holistic care, and as entrepreneurs. For a description of the variety of career choices for nurses, see *301 Careers in Nursing* (Fitzpatrick, Ea, & Bai, 2017).[8] This book—a virtual nursing career

Table 12.1

Industries With the Highest Levels of Employment for RNs

Industry	Employment (%)
General medical and surgical hospitals	30.62
Outpatient care centers	15.38
Home healthcare services	12.50
Skilled nursing facilities	9.51
Offices of physicians	7.63

Sources: Data from U.S. Bureau of Labor Statistics. (n.d.-a). *Occupational outlook handbook.* Retrieved from https://www.bls.gov/ooh/healthcare/registered-nurses.htm; U.S. Bureau of Labor Statistics. (n.d.-a). *Registered nurses.* Retrieved from https://data.bls.gov/cgi-bin/print.pl/oes/current/oes291141.htm

BOX 12.1 HIGHEST PAYING NURSING JOBS

1. Certified registered nurse anesthetist
2. General nurse practitioner
3. Gerontological nurse practitioner
4. Pain management nurse
5. Psychiatric nurse practitioner
6. Certified nurse midwife
7. Family nurse practitioner
8. Informatics nurse
9. Clinical nurse specialist
10. Nursing administrator
11. Nursing educator
12. Neonatal nurse
13. Critical care nurse
14. Health policy nurse
15. Medical-surgical nurse

"encyclopedia"—describes numerous positions that nurses can aspire to and lists required education, core competencies and skills, and related resources for researching positions.

CAREER OPPORTUNITIES FOR NURSES

Opportunities for nurses are endless, in both direct care and leadership roles. In the past, direct care nurses were hired into clinical nurse ("staff nurse") roles and could essentially remain in that type of role for most of their careers. Beginning in the 1970s, clinical ladders were introduced to allow nurses to advance within direct care roles. The next section explores avenues for advancement as a direct care nurse or a nurse leader.

Direct Care Nurse Advancement

Advancement for direct care nurses is typically provided through clinical ladder programs (CLPs) that are hospital based. CLPs were instituted in the 1970s to recognize and reward direct care nurses, promote nurse satisfaction, and enhance recruitment and retention. A CLP entails meeting requirements such as attainment of a BSN or advanced degree, precepting other nurses, obtaining a specialty certification, serving on committees, and conducting evidence-based performance improvement (PI) projects and research. Benefits of completing a rung on a clinical ladder usually include a sense of accomplishment and self-fulfillment, an increase in earnings, an advanced title (e.g., from Clinical Nurse I to Clinical Nurse II), and recognition in internal publications. CLPs are usually managed by the nursing and human resources departments.

An exemplar of CLPs is one sponsored by NewYork-Presbyterian Hospital (NYPH) in New York. Initiated in the early 2000s, the NYPH CLP provides for autonomy by allowing nurses to select from a list of professional development projects to meet requirements. The process begins with meeting eligibility criteria, successfully completing requirements specified in the application, and ends with a Clinical Ladder Committee review and approval. Following initial advancement on the clinical ladder, a nurse must meet renewal requirements at prescribed intervals to remain at the advanced level. The CLP at NYPH promotes self-actualization and recognition for direct care nurses.

Advancement to Leadership Roles

For nurses who want to pursue a management or leadership position, a CLP is a great place to start. In addition, leadership development programs that are focused on enhancing management and leadership skills also exist in some hospitals. These programs are usually managed by talent management professionals who are part of the human resources department. Talent management professionals are trained in the use of tools such as personal and behavioral style assessments such as DiSC° and Myers-Briggs, 360-degree feedback, and job fit inventories, to name a few. Some hospitals also have formal processes in place such as succession planning to ensure that there are nurses in the pipeline to fill vacant leadership positions created by attrition, and high potential leadership programs aimed at preparing selected nurses for management and leadership positions.

PREPARING FOR YOUR CAREER ADVANCEMENT

"Ask for what you want and be prepared to get it."

—Maya Angelou

When opportunities present themselves, be prepared to step up to the challenge! That includes something as simple as having a résumé that is up to date and best reflects your current accomplishments. We cannot always time when good things will happen to us, so having the tools that you need to take advantage of opportunities should be a priority. You owe it to yourself to be ready when an opportunity presents itself! The following steps toward preparedness have proven to be helpful to me and many successful nurses I have met during my career journey.

Step 1: Take Stock of What You Want and Where You Might "Fit In"

Choosing a position that you feel may advance your career is not just about finding one where the job description fits your experience. A careful assessment of what you value is a good place to start to determine if you will thrive in your next role. The book *Balance for Busy People: Managing Your Health, Money, Time, Space, and Relationships*[9] (Russ, 2001) includes a Values Inventory (Exhibit 12.1) that will help you determine what motivates you and offers clues to what you should look for in a career opportunity. I have included it here as a tool that you can use to assess your values.

Exhibit 12.1

Values Inventory

Instructions: Check off 10 values that are most important to you. Make sure the ones you check are ones that actually guide your actions on a daily basis. The list is by no means a complete list of all possible values and are not in order of importance.

___safety	___community service
___equality	___financial security
___strong work ethic	___quality
___power	___health
___reputation	___ambition
___spirituality	___justice
___accomplishments	___philanthropy
___creativity	___love
___family	___orderliness
___honesty	___selflessness
___life	___productivity
___self-esteem	___humility
___relationships	___respect
___altruism	___loyalty
___trustworthiness	___integrity
___sincerity	___leisure

You can prioritize the ten values you chose down to five to make your decision-making about a career option or opportunity more realistic. There may be few opportunities that meet all of your top ten values. An organization's vision, mission, and values statements will offer insights into what the organization is all about, but asking the right questions during the interview process can be more insightful, such as:

1. *How would you describe the culture here, and how is the culture "lived" on a daily basis?*
2. *Can you tell me any real-life stories about the culture in the organization and in the department?*
3. *What are the top three reasons that nurses leave employment in the organization and in the department?*
4. *What opportunities exist for nurses to make meaningful (measurable) contributions?*

A customized mission statement for your career journey and your personal life can be created using the Values Inventory. Formats for mission statements can be found in the literature and on the Internet. One that I found helpful is a format created by FranklinCovey. To view a sample of a mission statement, see *Balance for Busy People: Managing Your Health, Money, Time, Space, and Relationships*[9] (Russ, 2001).

An important aspect of finding where you "fit in" is determining personal characteristics that can enhance your career success or areas that are opportunities for improvement. Examples of tools that can offer insights into personal characteristics, styles, and or behavior patterns are the Myers-Briggs Type Inventory (MBTI) and DiSC. The MBTI provides an assessment of where you prefer to focus your energy, how you take in information, how you prefer to make decisions, and how you view the outer world. The MBTI has a career version for assessing what careers best suit you based on your personal style. The DiSC tool describes behavior patterns. Both MBTI and DiSC are best administered by trained facilitators who may be part of your human resources or talent management department.

Another useful tool for self-assessment is the SWOT analysis. The letters S-W-O-T stand for strengths, weaknesses, opportunities, and threats. Invented by in the 1960s by Albert Humphrey, a management consultant at the Stanford Research Institute, SWOT analysis can provide an assessment of where you may need to focus your attention when deciding on a career opportunity. When developing a SWOT, keep in mind that strengths and weaknesses are internal, that is, more easily controlled by you, and opportunities and threats are external and are not generally under your control. Opportunities are external events or areas that you can *capitalize on* or *take advantage of* and *not* areas of weakness. The beauty of the SWOT analysis is it can be used as a personal tool and a business tool. Business uses of SWOT include gathering information to make decisions such as where to focus marketing and sales efforts.

Step 2: Take Advantage of Professional Development Opportunities

Obtain a BSN or Advanced Degree

In October 2010, the Institute of Medicine (IOM), the health arm of the National Academy of Sciences, recommended that by the year 2020, 80% of nurses have a baccalaureate degree and that nurses practice to the full extent of their education and training. Other recommendations made by the IOM were:

- Academic progression for nurses should be seamless.
- Nurses should be full partners with physicians and other healthcare professionals in redesigning healthcare in the United States (IOM, 2010).

These recommendations have been promoted by organizations such as the ANCC, which has incorporated the promotion of lifelong learning for nurses into the Journey to Magnet Excellence' standards. Most hospitals have done a great job of promoting higher education for nurses through tuition reimbursement programs that support nurses in their education endeavors.

Already have a BSN? Obtaining an advanced degree has been supported by more and more hospitals in terms of both providing flexible schedules for nurses and providing more funding through tuition reimbursement. If you are interested in pursuing an advanced degree, most human resources departments can provide information on what the organization offers in terms of financial support and flexible schedules. It is important to look into your organization's affiliation agreements with local colleges to determine if your organization provides for clinical rotations or supports research projects, for example, for the school you choose to attend.

Want to pursue a master's degree? There are a variety of master's degrees in nursing, including those in nursing education, nursing administration, and health policy. Other advanced degrees that nurses hold include the master's in business administration and law degrees.

Interested in a terminal degree in nursing? Examples of these degrees include a PhD, DNSc, DNS, and DNP. The number of terminal degrees certainly requires that you do some research before choosing which one to pursue based on what career goals you want to pursue.

Obtain a Certification in Your Specialty

Obtaining a certification in your specialty is a great way to test your knowledge of your specialty and to remain current in your area of expertise. There are literally dozens of nationally recognized specialty certifications for nurses to choose from. The certification process entails taking a certification course, studying for the test utilizing specialty certification books, completing practice tests online, and sitting for the certification test at an authorized testing center. The first step is to decide which certification will benefit you the most in your career goals. Some nurses complete more than one certification. Examples of specialty certifications include:

- Acute critical care nurse
- Cardiac/vascular nurse
- Family nurse practitioner
- Gerontological nurse
- Informatics nurse
- Medical-surgical registered nurse
- Nurse executive
- Pain management nurse

For more nurse certifications, go to https://www.nursingworld.org, *the ANCC's website.*

Check with your employer to determine if reimbursement for testing and other types of support for certification are part of the menu of benefits. An increase in the hourly salary rate or a bonus may also be offered by some hospitals once certification is granted by the certifying agency (e.g., ANCC).

Choose a Mentor or Be a Mentor to a Nurse

Mentoring is a partnership between someone who may be experienced in areas such as leadership and interpersonal skills and a mentee, or protégé, who wants to develop those skill sets. The mentor's role is not to prescribe what a mentee should do, but rather to offer guidance and resources for the mentee to create a game plan for reaching preset goals. Being a mentor or a mentee is a great way to develop professionally. If you have never mentored someone, obtaining a mentor to assist you in your personal and professional development is a great way to "see how it's done." The mentoring relationship can be for a limited amount of time, usually a minimum of 6 months, but it can continue for a longer period of time—even years. A mentor can also be external to where you work. Some hospitals offer a formal mentoring program for those who want to become mentors. Mentoring programs usually include education and resources for guiding the relationship.

Benefits of mentoring include increased engagement for both mentor and mentee, decreased turnover, and advantages for nurses who may be placed in the pipeline when a management or leadership position opens. The process of becoming a mentor includes the completion of a mentoring education program, development of a contract between mentor and mentee so that logistics and expectations are understood, and provision for documentation of mentoring sessions, though some documentation may remain confidential. Logistics include agreements such as meeting frequency, time, and place and the methods of communication (in person, phone calls, and real-time social media platforms). A mentoring contract may include, in addition to logistics, the time frame for the relationship and a format for goal setting, such as the SMART (**S**pecific, **M**easurable, **A**chievable, **R**elevant, and **T**imebound) goals methodology. The SMART goals methodology will be discussed,later in this chapter.

Regarding choosing a mentor for yourself, mentors can provide guidance for both your professional and personal lives. I have had mentors during most of my career, and they have assisted me in navigating roles during my tenure with an employer and in pursuing external opportunities.

Become a Preceptor

Being a preceptor to a new nurse or experienced nurse new to your organization enhances your awareness of practicing in evidence-based ways. Let's face it, in any profession, after several years of practicing in the profession, the way we practice may change based on what we know works versus what is recommended by evidence-based practices (EBPs) and policy. When I was a preceptor for new hires during my career, I felt an obligation to consult available resources when teaching them the ropes. Resources included policies and procedures, pharmacy-based literature, and Lippincott⁺, to name a few. Precepting was, by far, one of the most rewarding professional development initiatives that I took part in as a direct care nurse. It afforded me the opportunity to "up my game" and to pass on knowledge and skills that are evidence based. More importantly, precepting gave me the opportunity to make new hires comfortable with the care they delivered. I recall how nervous I was when I gave my first injection as a new grad! Today, the benefits of precepting include an increase in pay in some healthcare organizations and may fulfill a requirement for advancement on a CLP. Preceptor programs are usually managed by the professional development or education department in collaboration with nurse managers and leaders.

Join a Committee or Work Group

Committees are in abundance in most healthcare organizations. While this is the case, you should not join a committee or work group without: (a) determining a valid purpose for joining and (b) making a commitment to be engaged. You may also be "assigned" to be part of a committee, but if that is the case, commitment is still part of the deal. A committee you've been assigned to may turn out to be one of the best professional development opportunities in your career. Common committees in healthcare organizations include infection control, safety, quality, nurse practice, and research. There are also nursing leadership committees that offer excellent opportunities for you to utilize leadership skills and to enhance communication skills. Committee leadership or membership may also provide opportunities to participate in subcommittee work that can lead to your participation in presentations on process improvements, patient care improvements, and patient experience enhancements.

Participate in Shared Governance Groups

Instituted in healthcare over 30 years ago, shared governance (SG) provides for greater professional autonomy for nurses and empowers nurses to take more responsibility for their practice. SG is a shared decision-making model based on principles of partnership, equity, accountability, and ownership at the point of service (Haag-Heitmann & George, 2010). The governing group, usually a nursing unit–based or a department-based council comprised of a majority of direct care nurses, is responsible for identifying projects to effect positive changes in nurse practice, the nurse practice environment, and patient care outcomes. SG meetings are held on an ongoing periodic basis and follow Roberts' Rules of Order to ensure that proceedings are efficient and effective and involve active participation from its members. SG council membership usually consists of a chair and co-chair who assume the responsibility of leading meetings. Decisions of the council are made based by consensus, meaning whatever the group decides, *everyone* will act as a champion for the decision, whether they were for it or against it.

The beauty of SG is direct care nurses are in control of council business and are able to use their expertise as direct care nurses to impact positive change. The nurse manager or nurse leader acts as an occasional ad hoc guest and can lend support and resources to the council as needed. Membership on a unit council is a great way to enhance your leadership skills or participate in improvement initiatives that make a measurable difference. Examples of projects that unit councils may spearhead include the implementation of new practices or the revision of practices that are evidence based, such as falls protocols and pressure ulcer reduction initiatives. Results are presented as reductions in the rate of such events, and data expressed as a rate are readily available from the organization's quality department. Unit council projects provide opportunities for presentation to organization-wide groups, and these presentations can be added to your list of accomplishments on a résumé.

Join a Professional Organization

Membership in a professional organization is a great way to enhance your knowledge about the nursing profession and nursing specialties. Professional organizations also provide opportunities to serve on committees both as a leader or as a member and to take part in projects that advance the profession. Most nursing professional organizations also provide opportunities for you to participate in community events such as health fairs and organized walks to benefit health-related charities. The cost for joining a professional nursing organization is usually affordable and offers discounts for conferences, publications, products, and services. Membership fees and attendance at conferences may also be reimbursed by your employer. Other benefits offered by membership-based organizations include access to:

- The organization's publications
- Local, regional, national, and even international professional development events
- Networking opportunities (professional and personal)
- Best practices from other organizations (poster and podium presentations)
- Opportunities to showcase your and your organization's work (e.g., poster and podium presentations)
- Career advancement opportunities

Examples of nursing organizations and the websites of those organizations are listed in Table 12.2.

Table 12.2

Nursing Organizations

Organization	Website
American Nurses Association	www.nursingworld.org
Academy of Medical-Surgical Nurses	www.amsn.org
American Academy of Nurse Practitioners	www.aanp.org
American Academy of Ambulatory Care Nursing	www.aaacn.org
American Association of Critical-Care nurses	www.aacn.org
American College of Nurse Midwives	www.midwife.org
American Psychiatric Nurses Association	www.apna.org
American Organization of Nurse Executives	www.aone.org
American Forensics Nurses	www.amrn.com
American Association of Legal Nurse Consultants	www.aalnc.org
Association for Nursing Professional Development	www.anpd.org
Home Healthcare Nurses Association	www.hhna.org
Sigma Theta Tau, International Honor Society of Nursing	www.nursingsociety.org
Society of Gastroenterology Nurses and Associates	www.sgna.org

Participate in Conferences and Workshops

As stated in the "Join a Professional Organization" section of this chapter, one of the benefits of joining a professional organization is discounts to conferences sponsored by the organization. I recently attended the American Psychiatric Nurses Association/New York chapter's annual conference. This conference included well-delivered presentations by experts in the field of psychiatric nursing and related topics. Expenses for this one-day conference were reasonable, including conference registration, travel, and hotel accommodations for one night. The point is, great educational opportunities don't have to involve great expense.

One of the responsibilities of nurses who attend conferences and workshops is to share the information with nurse peers and leaders when they return. If there is no formal process at your organization for sharing what you take away from an educational event, you can simply present a brief synopsis of what was presented as well as ideas for best practices that your organization can implement after proper vetting and approval. Implementation of a best practice that you present after attending a conference is a great accomplishment to add to your résumé and to include in your portfolio. Building a portfolio is discussed later in this chapter.

Volunteer to Participate in Projects

Examples of projects include PI, EBP, and research. All three of these types of projects can be unit or organization based, and all can originate in a SG unit council. All three have specific methodologies associated with them and vary in terms of time commitment and capabilities. The following is a summary of each.

- *PI* initiatives may take the least time and usually employ a methodology such as Plan-Do-Study-Act (PSDA) or Plan-Do-Check-Act (PDCA), which provides a template for steps from beginning to end. Examples of topics that may lend themselves to the PDSA methodology are falls reduction on a unit and reducing catheter-associated urinary tract infections. PDSA can also be used for process modification to improve efficiency in care delivery. DMAIC is another PI methodology. Steps for DMAIC are (a) define the problem, (b) measure, (c) analyze the cause of the problem, (d) improve, and (e) control (or monitor the impact of the change).
- EBP initiatives usually take more time and follow a process, including formulation of a question, a review of the literature, evaluation of what is found in the literature, implementation of a new practice or change in an existing practice, and evaluation of the new practice or change in practice.
- *Research* usually takes more time than PI and EBP and may entail a well-designed research question and hypothesis, a review

of the literature, and statistical analysis of data. The nursing research department in your organization can assist you with the development of a research project from beginning to end. In some organizations, the completion of a research education program is a requirement for conducting research, and some research studies require institutional review board approval. A preliminary discussion with your research committee or department is a good place to start your research endeavors.

Publish an Article

Whether you have been a nurse for two decades or two years, there are topics that you can write about with confidence. If you have been in the profession for a number of years, topics you can write about include clinical ones and ones based on your roles in management and leadership. If you are a new grad or novice nurse, you can write about your experiences as a new grad or novice and your acclimation to nursing and the new role you are in—including inspiring stories about your first position as a nurse. Testimonial articles are great for motivating nurses who are in the same career stage as you. And articles don't have to be lengthy to be accepted by a publication, whether an internal one or external one. I remember writing a short, two-page article for *Nursing Management* magazine when I was in the early stages of my career. I was ecstatic when I received notice that it was going to be published!

Take Continuing Education Courses

Continuing education courses provided by your employer or an outside company are convenient and are an easy way to enhance your skills, expertise, and knowledge about a wide variety of topics. Topics can range from clinical topics to how to manage difficult conversations. Some courses offered by healthcare organizations focus on personal health and well-being at no cost to you. Other courses offered, usually online, provide contact hours that may be required for RN licensure renewal and/or a nationally recognized certification. These courses usually provide a certificate of completion—another document you can include in a portfolio.

Step 3: Build a Portfolio

As you begin to participate in career growth opportunities like some of the ones mentioned in Step 2, the results of your participation are potentially significant events to document in your journal and to add to a portfolio of your work. Portfolios are useful for illustrating your accomplishments in black and white. They are useful in creating a kind of "show and tell" and illustrate experiences and accomplishments outlined in your résumé. Part of building a portfolio is keeping track of your accomplishments, lessons learned, and thoughts and feelings about what happens in your life and at work. Journaling is a great way to capture important events in real time. Journaling is both an objective and subjective activity—cataloging what actually occurred *and* the feelings and perceptions you had during and after events. I am a big proponent of journaling as it provides benefits that we may not realize at first. Some of benefits of journaling include:

1. It is a method of cataloging events that you may forget about as time passes.
2. It is a record of major milestones in your life and your career.
3. Events written in a journal can provide information that you can add to a résumé, performance review, and portfolio.
4. It provides a way of "letting go" of events that are/were problematic.
5. It is a source of motivation when things are going well or are not progressing according to your plans.
6. It creates spontaneous smiling and sometimes laughing at events that you may have forgotten about.

As stated earlier, journaling can provide information for updating your résumé. Journal entries may include notes about patient care and patient experience projects you facilitated or were part of, policies and procedures you assisted in revising or creating, process improvements you facilitated in your department, team building activities you facilitated, and financial stewardship projects that you led. When you are ready to create your résumé or update it, consider the following tips for enhancing this important part of your portfolio:

- Utilize a template, as a template makes it easier to decide what content to include. If you decide not to use a template, make sure that your résumé is categorized and headers such as experience, education, and awards and honors are highlighted.
- There are two basic types of résumés, including functional and chronological, although the two styles can be combined. Functional résumés focus on skills and experience, while chronological résumés focus on the positions you have held. You may also target a résumé to a particular position you are applying for. If a résumé is the style that you choose to capture your experience, include as many measurable outcomes as possible (cost savings, improvement in patient experience scores, reduced turnover, etc.).
- A special format for presenting your experience is the curriculum vitae (CV). A CV details career experiences and includes academic pursuits such as publications, research, and awards and honors. CVs are used most often in academic settings.

- Ask for help when writing your résumé if you need it. Human resources and talent management professionals can assist you with creating a professional résumé. Some employers have leadership development programs and CLPs that include résumé writing as a component of these programs. If you decide to utilize the expertise of a résumé writer, be prepared to provide the writer with detailed information about your career. Most résumé writers will provide you with a form to complete prior to meeting with them that captures your experience.
- Review your résumé or CV for grammatical and spelling errors and print copies on good-quality paper.

While a journal can provide some of the information you need to create or update a résumé or CV, a professional portfolio should include documents that provide proof that what you stated in your résumé is accurately portrayed. Examples of documents you can consider including in your portfolio are:

- A résumé
- Diplomas for degrees
- Copies of certificates for nationally recognized certifications such as those administered by the ANCC and those that are skills based (Basic Life Support [BLS], Advanced Cardiovascular Life Support [ACLS], Crisis Prevention Intervention, etc.)
- Performance reviews
- Documentation of projects you led or participated in, including presentations, algorithms, and improved process flows
- Commendations, honors, awards, and thank-you letters
- Research project documentation
- Documentation of relevant continuing education programs (conference certificates, workshops, etc.)
- Personal style or behavioral style assessments that you are willing to share (*this can be a summary page included in the report if you don't want to share report details*)
- Books, articles, and other publications you authored or coauthored
- Conference participation, especially podium and poster presentations, and best practices implemented as a result of conference attendance

Portfolios can be electronic, but having a professional-looking hard copy of documents in some type of binder makes it easily accessible should the opportunity arise to present them. A few things to consider include avoiding the inclusion of documents that are proprietary and being sure to assess if the situation is right for presenting hard copies in meetings with potential employers.

Step 4: Set Goals for Charting Your Career Path

Your goals statements will provide a road map for getting to where you want to be in your career. If you plan to be on a nursing career path for decades or have been a nurse for a year or two, careful planning will generate enormous benefits for leading a self-actualizing work life. To create goals, start with information from the assessment tools you have at your disposal to determine your interests, values, personal and behavioral style, skills, competencies, and experience. Then take a look at the nursing career choices that exist. A good starting point is to refer to a resource such as *301 Careers in Nursing* (Fitzpatrick et al., 2017), a book that I mentioned earlier in this chapter. The next step is to create a list of three or four goals that you want to start with to move forward in your career. A methodology to create meaningful goals is the SMART methodology. Though the origin of SMART goals has been disputed by writers on the subject, the methodology has been around since the early 1980s and is helpful for achieving success in the attainment of personal and workplace goals. The SMART acronym, as noted earlier in the chapter, stands for **S**pecific, **M**easurable, **A**chievable, **R**elevant, and **T**imebound. Questions to consider when using SMART are:

1. *Specific: Is the goal specific, that is, is it simple and meaningful?*
2. *Measurable: How will I know that I have been successful in achieving the goal?*
3. *Achievable: Is the goal attainable?*
4. *Relevant: Is the goal reasonable and realistic?*
5. *Timebound: Is there a deadline?*

As you can see from the example in Table 12.3, the SMART methodology is a sort of "litmus test" for determining if your goals are clear, concise, and important. Vague goals such as "I want to become a better nurse" are a lot harder to wrap your arms around and are harder, if not impossible, to measure. To make goals easier to manage, you can create no more than one or two SMART goals to achieve in the first 6 months of the year and one or two in the remaining 6 months of the year.

Develop a Plan for Achieving Goals

Action planning, while not the final step in meeting goals, is a big step in preparing for upward movement in your career. Projects and other actions that you complete on your action plan are ones you can include on a résumé or CV and in your portfolio. A word of caution is to be sure to streamline the action plan to include only those actions that directly relate to the goal you want to accomplish. Exhibit 12.2 is an example of an action plan for achieving the SMART goal in the previous section.

Table 12.3

Specific, Measurable, Achievable, Relevant, and Timebound (SMART) Goal Example

SMART Goal	Specific?	Measurable?	Achievable?	Relevant?	Timebound?
Obtain a nationally recognized certification in psychiatric nursing by June 2022.	Yes *Obtaining a certification is meaningful: Certification provides knowledge about my specialty and will keep me up to date in my area of expertise; it is also meaningful because it is a requirement for my future pursuit of becoming a Clinical Nurse I.*	Yes *At the end of certification testing, I will receive a letter stating that I passed, and this will be followed by an official certificate that I can attach to my CLP application.*	Yes *The certification prep course is available at my hospital, and the cost for the program and testing will be reimbursed. I have the time to take the certification review course. I can devote 2 hours a week to studying for the test for a few weeks before testing.*	Yes *Enhancing my knowledge of psychiatric nursing will enable me to become aware of the most current best practices in my specialty.*	Yes *I have set a goal for obtaining my certification by June 2022.*

CLP, clinical ladder program.

Exhibit 12.2

Action Plan for Achieving the SMART Goal

SMART Goal: Obtain a nationally recognized certification in psychiatric nursing by June 2022

Action	Deadline	Resources	Date Completed
1. Register for the December 2021 psychiatric nursing certification review course	By 10/31/21	Continuing education policy and procedure, continuing education request form, and online registration	
2. Take certification review course	December 2021	n/a	
2. Register for certification test	by 12/15/21	Online registration	
3. Schedule 2 hours/week to study notes for test and take online sample tests	Starting 3 weeks before testing date	ANCC psychiatric nursing certification review and resource book	
4. Take certification test	February 2022	Online registration for testing	

ANCC, American Nurses Credentialing Center.

SUCCESS STORY

Ophelia M. Byers, DNP, RN, WHNP-BC, RNC-OB, NEA-BC

Vice President, Patient Services, and Chief Nursing Officer, NewYork-Presbyterian Hudson Valley Hospital, New York

How long have you been an RN?

I have been an RN for 20 years, since July 1999.

Why did you decide to become an RN?

Three women have inspired my journey to and of nursing. Throughout my childhood, my maternal grandmother, Rachael Browne Singleton, proudly shared stories about her parents—especially her mother, Mary Washington Browne, who was also a "lay" or "granny" midwife in rural Georgia. My maternal great-grandmother provided care to women from the antepartum to postpartum phases and, according to family lore, attended the births of a few thousand babies. She also maintained a birth registry, and relatives still have her leather bag of clinical instruments and supplies. I shared my grandmother's immense pride in this family history and wanted to be like the phenomenal woman whom I would never meet, except through my grandmother's fond memories. I wanted to educate, empower, and provide clinical care for women throughout their life span. I wanted to be a midwife. I also wanted to be a nurse—to fulfill the dream my mother, Rheba Singleton, had for herself but exchanged for motherhood. Years later, when I started undergraduate study—after a year of "finding myself" and then joining the United States Army Reserves—I returned to the goals that would honor my great-grandmother, grandmother, mother, and myself. I started undergraduate study and began the journey to a nursing career in women and children's health.

What school did you attend to prepare you to become a nurse, and what advanced degrees and certifications do you hold?

For undergraduate study, I attended Rutgers University, the branch campus in my hometown of Camden, New Jersey. There I earned a BSN.

For postgraduate study, I attended Stony Brook University in New York and earned an MSN. I did not train to be a nurse midwife as I once aspired, but instead I studied to be a women's health nurse practitioner to provide outpatient obstetric and gynecologic care. For my DNP, I attended Case Western Reserve University in Ohio, and in partnership with the National Black Nurses Association, my scholarly research was on racism-related stress and psychological resilience in Black/African American nurses.

I have earned, and currently maintain, the following national certifications from the National Certification Corporation (NCC): Women's Health Nurse Practitioner, Board Certified (WHNP-BC), Inpatient Obstetrics (RNC-OB), and the Electronic Fetal Monitoring subspecialty certification (C-EFM). I earned, and maintain, the following national certification from the American Nurses Credentialing Center: Nurse Executive Advanced, Board Certified (NEA-BC).

Where was your first job as a nurse, and how did you get the job?

My first job as a RN was on the Children's Rehab Hospital (CRH) Pediatrics unit of Thomas Jefferson University Hospital (TJUH) in Philadelphia, Pennsylvania. Years prior, the brick-and-mortar CHR in another Pennsylvania city had closed down and was condensed into a small unit within TJUH. The unit was like a step-down for babies who graduated from the level IIIC neonatal intensive care unit but were not stable enough to go home.

How did one who aspired to care for obstetric patients end up with a first nursing job caring for sick babies?

A nurse externship. My senior year of nursing school, I earned a paid externship on CRH Pediatrics. I was educated, empowered, and embraced by one of the most clinically astute, cohesive, and fun teams of nurses I've ever had the privilege to work with. Every single day, being at work was like being at home; and it was a no-brainer, for the team and me, that I would work there for my first professional nursing role. I don't recall interviewing for the role, though I'm sure it happened. However, I vividly recall is something I've carried in my soul my whole career thus far: A couple of the nurses who had become great work friends—more like big sisters—invited me into one of the three multicrib rooms on the small unit, sat me down, and said, "You've got the job, and we're proud of you. Now, don't get cocky."

Did you/do you have a mentor and/or coach?

I have been fortunate to have leaders who invested in me and mentored me, often purposely and sometimes unwittingly. I have benefited from being an observer of people and a student of experiences. I ingest various views, styles, beliefs, truths, kudos, and criticisms. Then, I metabolize what I have learned, taking only what I need to grow and develop. This approach has allowed me to learn from many different people's rich experiences and perspectives, not just those of one person with a specific professional profile. This approach to intrapersonal cultivation has been a significant part of my career success.

How have personal assessment tools benefited you in your career?

In my management roles, I have completed the following leadership assessments: Myers-Briggs, DiSC®, and the Korn Ferry Four Dimensions of Executive (K4FD-Exec) Assessment. In my functional leader role, I have also received 360-degree feedback. All the assessments—particularly for leadership profile or style—had common threads and were mostly accurate in my strengths and vulnerabilities as a leader. I used all assessment outcomes and recommendations to bolster my confidence in what I was doing well and to focus my efforts on my areas for improvement.

What role have professional organizations played in your career?

- Sigma Theta Tau (STT)
- American Nurses Association (ANA)
- Nurse Practitioners in Women's Health (NPWH)
- Association of Women's Health, Obstetric and Neonatal Nurses (AWHONN)
- American Organization for Nursing Leadership (AONL)
- Kids Creative (board member and chair of the board's Audit and Risk Committee)

Though these organizations vary in focus, they have an overarching goal: promoting and improving health and wellness. Participation in these organizations has made me a better person and professional by exposing me to new people and innovations and evidence-based approaches in clinical care and, as important, enlightening me about efforts outside of the healthcare industry that could be transformative if adopted by healthcare.

What role has networking played in your career?

Intentional, goal-inspired professional networking is a skill that I have not yet honed. Certainly I enjoy meeting new people and sustaining meaningful connections; however, a growth opportunity for me is to use networking more often. I currently don't use these opportunities as often as I could, which aligns with the "extroverted introvert" assessment of my personal style on the Myers-Briggs personal style inventory. Making more room for mutually beneficial professional relationships is a personal goal, that is, to be willing and able to enlist resources from others just as I am willing to give my time, energy, and ideas to support their efforts.

What are the top three highlights of your career?

The first of the top three highlights of my career is becoming licensed as a registered professional nurse—after being the first of my maternal grandparents' progeny to graduate from college. This honors my mother, and her dreams and sacrifices. The second highlight is the first time I cared for a family during labor and birth of their baby, which honors my great-grandmother, the lay midwife, and one of her proud children, my grandmother. The third, and most recent, highlight is earning the role of vice president of patient services and chief nursing officer. This attainment is one my forebears had not envisioned, perhaps did not know existed, but their insistence that, with each generation, views expand wider, dreams grow bigger, goals aim higher, and empowerment runs deeper has been the driving force of my career. Their commitment to helping others—whether as clinical caregivers or mothers—has been my inspiration for being the best nurse and the best leader I can be. Most importantly, this career highlight honors my immediate family: my husband Charles, our daughter Haile Sarafina, and our son Charles Ayinde. I entered leadership practice when Haile was an infant and Charles not yet born. In the 11-year period since, I served in six leadership roles, and all were progressive management roles except for one functional leadership role that allowed me the schedule flexibility to care for a toddler and newborn. The rigor and pace of my career would not have been possible without my husband and children's support, patience, resilience, and shared commitment to our family bond. Indeed, "it takes a village . . ."

Chart your career path from start to finish.

After becoming a licensed RN, I became a clinical nurse on a pediatrics unit in a Pennsylvania hospital. I then became a travel nurse and completed over 15 assignments in various U.S. hospitals and in myriad pediatric specialties. Next, I settled in New York to take a permanent clinical nurse role and become a labor and delivery (L&D) nurse. My charge nurse experiences whet my appetite for formal leadership, and I became an assistant nurse manager and then a nurse manager. Later, to finally be able to work at a hospital I long admired (and to better meet the demands of co-parenting a toddler and infant), I left the nurse manager role to take a functional leadership role as a patient safety nurse in obstetrics. Once I regained some semblance of personal–professional equilibrium, I returned to the management realm, taking a patient care director (nurse manager) role, the same level of management I had been in before the functional leader role. From patient care director, I became a director of nursing, and from director of nursing, I became VP of patient services and CNO. I look forward to learning, leading, and serving in this essential healthcare executive role; and I am resolute and excited that the end of my career remains unwritten.

CONCLUSION

Nursing is a respected profession that has created a wealth of opportunities for those of us who practice it. Based on predictions about future trends in healthcare, nursing will continue to be a profession that attracts tens of thousands to it. For today's nurses, hospitals provide only one of many places where they can pursue career *opportunities* that are compatible with their values, personal styles, educational preparation, and skill sets. Nurses who invest in planning a career path for themselves are in the best position to take advantage of opportunities when they are presented.

Key Points

- Career opportunities for nurses are boundless. Many options remain for both direct care and leadership roles.
- Advancing in your career requires commitment to being involved in organizational initiatives, your professional organization, and continuing education.
- Setting a SMART goal helps ensure your success in achieving your personal vision.

References

American Nurses Credentialing Center. (2017). *2019 Magnet® application manual.* Silver Spring, MD: American Nurses Credentialing Center.
Brenan, M. (2019, August 5). *Nurses again outpace other professions for honesty, ethics.* Retrieved from https://news.gallup.com/poll/245597/nurses-again-outpace-professions-honesty-ethics.aspx

Fitzpatrick, J. J., Ea, E. E., & Bai, L. S. (2017). *301 careers in nursing.* New York, NY: Springer Publishing Company.

Haag-Heitmann, B., & George, V. (2010). *Guide for establishing shared governance: A starter's toolkit.* Sliver Spring, MD: American Nurses Credentialing Center.

Institute of Medicine. (2011). *The future of nursing: Leading change, advancing health (Rep.).* Washington, DC: National Academies Press.

McMenamin, P. (2016, June). *ANA's nurses by the Numbers™* (p. 8).

Nurse.org. (n.d.). *15 highest paying nursing careers* [Infographic]. Retrieved from https://nurse.org/articles/15-highest-paying-nursing-careers

Russ, A. M. (2001). *Balance for busy people: Managing your health, money, time, space, and relationships* (pp. 109–111). Miami, FL: Russ Consulting.

U.S. Bureau of Labor Statistics. (n.d.-a). *Occupational outlook handbook.* Retrieved from https://www.bls.gov/ooh/healthcare/registered-nurses.htm

U.S. Bureau of Labor Statistics. (n.d.-b). *Registered nurses.* Retrieved from https://data.bls.gov/cgi-bin/print.pl/oes/current/oes291141.htm

Additional Resources

Cardillo, D. W. (2018). *The ultimate career guide for nurses: Practical advice for thriving at every stage of your career.* Silver Spring, MD: American Nurses Association.

Duffield, C., Baldwin, R., Roche, M., & Wise, S. (2013). Job enrichment: Creating meaningful career development opportunities for nurses. *Journal of Nursing Management, 22*(6), 697–706. doi:10.1111/jonm.12049

Marshall, L. (2010). *Take charge of your nursing career: Open the door to your dreams.* Indianapolis, IN: Sigma Theta Tau International.

Mind Tools. (n.d.). *SMART goals—How to make your goals achievable.* Retrieved from https://www.mindtools.com/pages/article/smart-goals.htm

Phillips, J. M., & Boivin, J. (2014). *Accelerate your career in nursing: A guide to professional advancement and recognition.* Indianapolis, IN: Sigma Theta Tau International.

Watts, M. D. (2010). Certification and clinical ladder as the impetus for professional development. *Critical Care Nursing Quarterly, 33*(1), 52–59. doi:10.1097/cnq.0b013e3181c8e333

Index

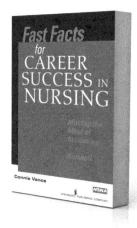
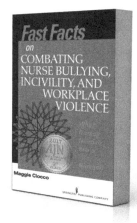
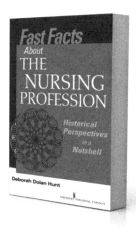
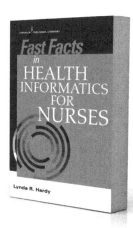

Printed in the United States
by Baker & Taylor Publisher Services